UNDERSTANDING VITAMINS AND MINERALS

The Prevention Total Health System®

UNDERSTANDING VITAMINS AND MINERALS

by the Editors of
Prevention® Magazine

 Rodale Press, Emmaus, Pennsylvania

Library of Congress Cataloging in Publication Data
Main entry under title:

Understanding vitamins and minerals.

(The Prevention total health system)
Includes bibliographical references and index.
    1. Vitamins in human nutrition—Addresses, essays, lectures. 2. Minerals in human nutrition—Addresses, essays, lectures. 3. Dietary supplements—Addresses, essays, lectures. I. Prevention (Emmaus, Pa.) II. Series.
QP771.U63 1983   613.2′8   83-21282
ISBN 0-87857-463-8 hardcover
    4 6 8 10 9 7 5   hardcover

The Prevention Total Health System®
Series Editors: William Gottlieb, Mark Bricklin
Understanding Vitamins and Minerals Editors:
    William Gottlieb, Carol Keough
Writers: Sharon Faelten, Jim Nechas, Stephen
    Williams, Marian Wolbers
Research Chief: Carol Baldwin
Assistant Research Chief, Prevention Health Books:
    Christy Kohler
Researchers: Holly Clemson, Susan Nastasee, Joann
    Williams, Martha Capwell, Pam Mohr, Carole
    Rapp, Nancy Smerkanich
Art Director: Karen A. Schell
Associate Art Director: Jerry O'Brien
Art Production Manager: Jane C. Knutila
Designers: Lynn Foulk, Alison Lee
Illustrators: Bascove, Susan M. Blubaugh, Joe Lertola
Project Assistants: Tom Chinnici, Linda Jacopetti,
    John Pepper
Director of Photography: T. L. Gettings
Photography Coordinator: Margaret Skrovanek
Photographic Stylists: Renee Grimes, Kay Seng
    Lichthardt, Kathryn E. Sommons, J. C. Vera
Photo Librarian: Shirley S. Smith
Staff Photographers: Christopher Barone, Carl Doney,
    T. L. Gettings, John P. Hamel, Mitchell T. Mandel,
    Margaret Skrovanek, Christie C. Tito,
    Sally Shenk Ullman
Copy Editor: Jane Sherman
Production Manager: Jacob V. Lichty
Production Coordinator: Barbara A. Herman
Composite Typesetter: Brenda J. Kline
Production Assistant: Eileen Bauder
Office Personnel: Diana M. Gottshall, Susan Lagler,
    Carol Petrakovich, Cindy Harig, Marge Kresley,
    Donna Strubeck

Rodale Books, Inc.
Editorial Director: Carol Hupping
Managing Editor: William H. Hylton
Copy Manager: Ann Snyder
Publisher: Richard M. Huttner
Director of Marketing: Eller Rama
Business Manager: Ellen J. Greene
Continuity Marketing Manager: John Taylor

Rodale Press, Inc.
Chairman of the Board: Robert Rodale
President: Robert Teufel
Executive Vice President: Marshall Ackerman
Group Vice Presidents: Sanford Beldon
                        Mark Bricklin
Senior Vice President: John Haberern
Vice Presidents: John Griffin
                  Richard M. Huttner
                  James C. McCullagh
                  Carol Hupping
                  David Widenmyer
Secretary: Anna Rodale

NOTICE

Contents

Preface   vii

Chapter 1: The Discovery of the Life Sparks   1

The vitamin pioneers battled scientific dogma and disdain to prove that *food* cures disease.

Chapter 2: Why You Need Food Supplements   11

Factory food, pollution, stress—they all drain you of nutrients. Here's how to plug the leak.

Chapter 3: Vitamin A—From A to Z   21

It seems hard to believe that one nutrient works in so many ways to guard health, but nature is rather adept at such miracles.

Chapter 4: The B Complex Vitamins   37

Together the B vitamins make up the roster of a winning nutritional team for health.

Chapter 5: Vitamin C: A Natural Ally   57

This nutrient has a knack for defending us in tough situations—from colds to cancer.

Chapter 6: Vitamin D Lets the Sun Shine In   75

This crucial vitamin strengthens your bones and nourishes your muscles and nerves.

Chapter 7: Vitamin E: Strong Medicine   81

Once the "vitamin in search of a deficiency," it's now lauded as a force that slows aging and strengthens the heart.

Chapter 8: Minerals: Foundation of Health   97

All the vitamins in the world do us little good without minerals.

Chapter 9: The Special Supplements   127

Our 4-star rating system is your guide to these unique health products.

Chapter 10: A Shopper's Guide to Supplements   145

Expert advice to help you choose supplements that are good for your body—and your budget.

Chapter 11: A Personal Supplement Program   153

This tailor-made nutritional guide shows how much of each vitamin and mineral *you* need.

Source Notes   164

Credits   165

Index   166

Full-Power Nutrition

Standing in a modern supermarket, it may appear inconceivable that anyone today could have a deficiency of vitamins or minerals. But appearances can be dangerously deceiving.

Consider, for instance, that about 25 percent of all the calories we average moderns eat come from added sugar, which contains nothing besides calories. Right off the bat, then, cross out one-fourth of our diet as a potential source of vitamins and minerals.

If we exclude those who never drink at all, those remaining take in, on the average, some 20 to 25 percent of all calories from alcohol. (Surprising, but that's what the most recent research says.) Alcoholic beverages contain at best only traces of vitamins and minerals. So between the sugar and the alcohol, our average person is now getting approximately *half* of his daily calorie quota from sources that are nutritional blanks.

Still more calories in a typical modern diet come from processed fats—table spreads, cooking fats, salad oils and fats added to baked goods. Such fats—which contain only a few traces of vitamins—may constitute another 15 to 30 percent of daily calories.

Put it all together and you can see that the same food technology that has given us the opportunity to eat like Roman emperors has also made it possible for us to waste two-thirds of our daily diets on food that couldn't keep a mouse alive.

Beyond mere existence, we know today that vitamins and minerals play a surprisingly important role in how we feel and perform. With no specific, classic symptoms of deficiency, for instance, we may still require more vitamins and minerals to clear up a skin problem, lift ourselves from depression or boost immunity from D-minus to A-plus.

Nothing, perhaps, is more fundamental to good health than full-power nutrition. And here is the place to learn about it: one of the key volumes in the Prevention Total Health System.®

Executive Editor, **Prevention**® Magazine

Preface

1

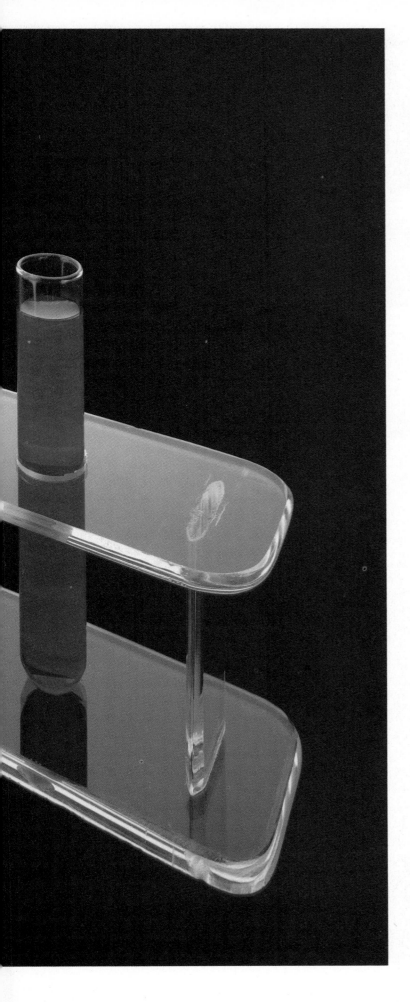

The Discovery of the Life Sparks

The vitamin pioneers battled scientific dogma and disdain to prove that *food* cures disease.

Bowed legs, scaled skin and enlarged hearts.

Vitamins can prevent these afflictions. Yet for years physicians and scientists prevented people from having vitamins.

This is the story of those years, years of prejudice, ignorance and blind hubris. Years when scientists in entrenched positions of medical orthodoxy rejected—in fact, even refused to test—the theories of the nutritional pioneers who realized that *food* can cure disease. That pellagra, beriberi, scurvy and rickets—killers and maimers of recent generations—all can be prevented by simple changes in diet. Their explanation was just too simple. But if they had been heeded, countless hunch-backed children would have stood straight, the ocean floor would be marked by fewer sailors' skeletons and American blacks would have suffered one less major indignity.

A PLAGUE OF CORN

"Nate, eat your mush," says Etta.

Nate spoons the gruel, leaving a small piece of fatback in the bowl to be savored at the end of the meal. The fatback is a treat. Etta has been serving Nate cornmeal mush with molasses every morning and night since time—or at least his memory—began.

Nate's body aches, but he knows it isn't from working all day in the cotton fields. It's a hollow ache, a cry, a hunger. The skin on his arms is dry and scaled like a sunburned lizard.

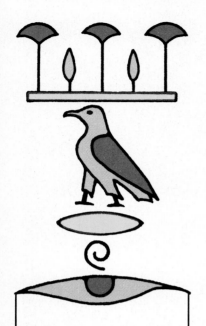

An Ancient Vitamin Cure

The column of drawings above is an Egyptian hieroglyphic—a type of ancient picture writing—that spells out "night blindness." And the suggested remedy seems as puzzling as the sphinx: beef liver cooked, squeezed, and placed against the eye.

But the folks who built the pyramids were on the right track; beef liver is a great source of vitamin A. Over 3,000 years later, modern scientists "discovered" that a lack of vitamin A causes night blindness.

John walks in and Nate knows there will be no peace this night. His father has been acting like a wild man lately. He doesn't drink—though he might if there were any money—but the way he acts makes the white men he works for call him just another crazy son of a slave. The cornmeal mush is killing the family. They have pellagra—but they couldn't give this sickness a name or tell you why they have it.

Scenes like these were repeated all over the South in the first part of this century. They won't happen again. The world now knows how easy it is to prevent pellagra—simply add the B vitamin niacin to the diet.

Pellagra is considered a "new" disease because it didn't occur until after Christopher Columbus brought the first corn plants to Europe from the New World. The Europeans saw corn as an easy-to-grow miracle crop and peasants began to depend on it for sustenance. That was the beginning of the end for many people. Whole communities were subject to the scales and dementia of pellagra. It is amazing that anything functioned where the workers were plagued by the dullness and persistent degeneration of their niacin-deficient bodies and minds.

Over the centuries, several people implicated diet as the cause of pellagra. Théophile Roussel, a French physician, showed that pellagra was associated with the poor and corn, and in 1848 convinced his government to discourage cultivation of the crop. As a result, the disease almost disappeared from France. But dependence on corn—and the resultant pellagra—continued in other countries, especially Italy, where outbreaks would occur every time the economy plunged and people were forced to eat almost nothing but corn.

Corn itself is not poisonous, of course. It is just incomplete. The niacin it contains is not easily metabolized by humans.

The Indians of the New World lived on corn-dependent diets for generations without any problems because they complemented corn with beans, squash, chilies and coffee, all sources of niacin. In Mexico the women added lime to corn after they ground it for tortillas, making the niacin in corn more available.

But pellagra victims—particularly those of the American South—ate bowl after bowl of cornmeal mush. During good times other foods were added, but they were rarely sufficient to counter the disease. The typical diet of the slaves and poor people was often referred to as the three-M diet: meat (actually just fatback), meal and molasses. This diet produced the four-D symptoms of pellagra: dermatitis, diarrhea, dementia—and finally, death.

Although many slaves suffered from pellagra, it was rarely officially diagnosed as such. It was called a "Negro disease" and "black tongue," and was at its worst during droughts or when farmers were particularly poor.

The three-M diet didn't change much as many blacks went from being slaves to being sharecroppers. In fact, pellagra was epidemic during the early 20th century, and 7,000 people died of the disease in 1928.

SOLVING THE MYSTERY

The first modern clue that pellagra was caused by diet came when the scientist Casimir Funk discovered that beriberi—another horrid disease—could be cured by what he called a *vitamine*, a substance in food. The beriberi vitamin that Funk discovered was thiamine (vitamin B_1). In the process, however, he also isolated niacin from rice polishings, but relegated it to the back shelf when he found that it didn't cure beriberi.

Another researcher, Carl Voegtlin, stated that pellagra was a deficiency disease, and criticized those who casually dismissed diet as a cause.

Finally, an open-minded and determined man was sent to the South by the U.S. government to get to the heart of the matter.

Joseph Goldberger toured small southern towns where men lay against the sides of shanties, listless and depressed from pellagra. Small children dressed in rags tugged at their mothers' hems, whimpering for relief from the painful sores that plagued them. And the women—until they were debilitated by hallucinations or

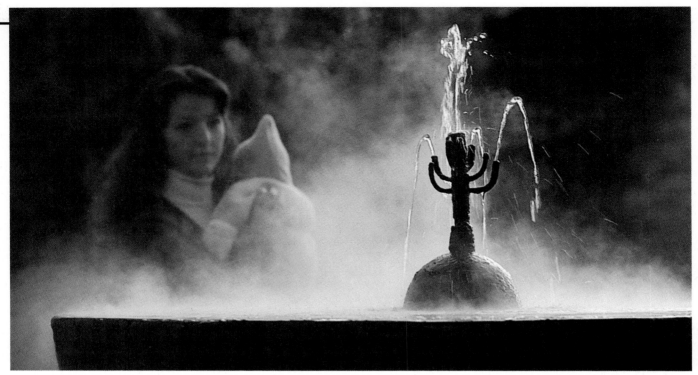

lack of energy—continued to cook corn: corn muffins, corn coffee, cornmeal mush and cornbread. It was all they could afford.

Goldberger was convinced that pellagra had a nutritional cause when he visited a public orphanage. He found the younger children typically bedridden and depressed, with severe sores. The older children, however, were fine. They were strong enough to work at odd jobs and pick up a little money, with which they bought fruit and vegetables to give life to their monotonous diet. Goldberger realized that Voegtlin had the right idea about the cure for pellagra: proper diet. To prove it, he arranged for *all* the children to get milk, meat and eggs. Within days, the youngsters who had previously dragged themselves through the days began to lift their heads and smile. At the orphanage, the outbreak of pellagra was over.

While Goldberger was solving the riddle, another government research team was exacerbating the problem. They announced that a certain species of fly was spreading the pellagra "microbe" with its sting. The public bought it, as did many physicians. Goldberger, desperate to let the truth be known about the disease that was affecting 170,000 people a year in the United States, took a great risk. He scraped red

scales from the idle legs of pellagra victims, mixed them with the foul excretions and mucus of the sick—and injected the substance into himself and his family. Then he ate some of it before shocked onlookers.

The family didn't get sick. The infection theory was swept aside.

Goldberger then induced pellagra in prison inmates in exchange for their early parole, and cured the disease with yeast, meat and milk. Goldberger didn't know what substance in food was needed to prevent pellagra, but he had proven that corn wasn't poisonous and that pellagra wasn't infectious.

It wasn't until 1937 that Conrad Elvehjem isolated the antipellagra nutrient. Much to the scientific community's surprise, it was Funk's early discovery—niacin.

POLISHED RICE, TARNISHED HEALTH

Between 1880 and 1883, over 6,000 men in the Japanese navy died from the paralysis, dementia and cardiac arrest that characterize beriberi.

In 1886, three sailors died. In 1887, none.

No vaccine was discovered. No microbe was controlled. Only the diet of the sailors was changed.

Kanekiro Takaki, a doctor with

Spring water—often laden with health-giving minerals—has been used as a source of natural medicine since long before there were doctors. This fountain channels the waters at Hot Springs National Park in Arkansas, where 5 million people visit every year. The park is the site of 47 springs, whose mineral-containing waters are used by health-seekers to relieve the tensions of modern life.

In an experiment conducted in 1907, young laboratory animals fed an artificial diet of lard, sugar and other substances failed to grow. But when F. G. Hopkins—a biochemist later awarded the Nobel Prize and called "the father of the vitamin theory"—added milk to their diets, the animals thrived. (Hopkins also conducted the experiment the other way around, taking milk away from the animals. On the artificial diet alone, the animals' growth was stunted.) After the experiment, Hopkins theorized that milk contained microscopic food factors essential for health. Scientists later chemically isolated those factors: the vitamins.

the Japanese navy, proved that a diet made up almost exclusively of polished rice was causing beriberi. Sailors on Japanese ships were plagued by the swaying, sheeplike walk and paralysis of the disease, but officers, whose diet was better, were rarely afflicted. So, after the naval ship *Riuyo* returned from a long cruise with 25 of its sailors dead and 144 sick with beriberi (out of a crew of 276), Takaki convinced the generally unresponsive naval commanders to let him experiment with another ship on an identical voyage. Takaki was convinced that beriberi was caused by an imbalance of carbon and nitrogen in the diet. He was wrong, but on the right track.

On the second ship, the sailors' normal diet, consisting primarily of rice, was replaced by a British diet including oatmeal, vegetables and condensed milk, a horrendous imposition on the highly ethnocentric Japanese. Fourteen sailors scoffed at the barbarous food and ate

primarily polished rice that they smuggled aboard. The ship returned and the 14 with the less adventurous taste buds were sick with beriberi. The rest were fine.

After that, shipboard rations were changed permanently and the death rate from beriberi dropped dramatically.

News of Takaki's findings reached unresponsive ears in Europe. His theories were seen as childish because they ignored germs. If only the Europeans had listened. The Dutch colonists in the Dutch East Indies (now Indonesia) would have been saved the expense of burying thousands of work gang members who found it difficult to labor with enlarged hearts and paralyzed legs.

And Dutch troops came down with beriberi so quickly in the field that they couldn't suppress native revolts in Northern Sumatra. In fact, the disease continued raging in the colonial empire until Christiaan Eijkman was sent by the Dutch to find out what *bacteria* was causing all the misery.

Eijkman had no success inducing beriberi in chickens by injecting them with "infectious blood," and almost gave up. But one day he looked outside and the whole flock was swaying crookedly around the courtyard. They had finally developed beriberi. And that was a surprise, because he had never tried to inject all the chickens in the flock, just a portion picked for the experiment. So why were they all sick?

There was no explanation until six months later, when the chickens showed a remarkable recovery. It turned out that they had been given expensive polished rice by a lazy kitchen worker and had developed beriberi. When a supervisor put the chickens back on the less expensive whole rice, the disease disappeared. The "refuse"—rice husks—was the cure.

Eijkman therefore took Takaki's conclusion one step further and said it was something in the polished rice that caused beriberi. Eijkman's arguments were flatly rejected by the authorities, who thought polished rice was a gift to the natives, and by scientists, who insisted that beriberi was caused by bacteria. The steam-

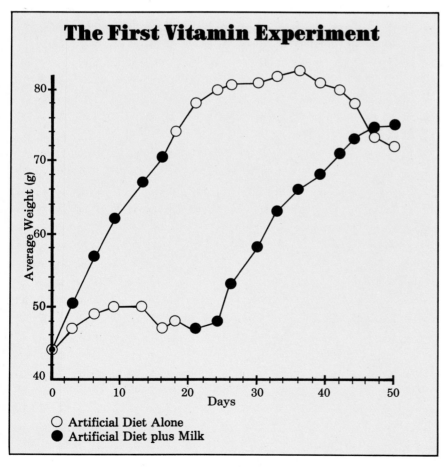

The First Vitamin Experiment

Average Weight (g)

○ Artificial Diet Alone
● Artificial Diet plus Milk

Days

powered rice mills that Westerners felt were civilizing the Far East were actually *causing* large-scale deaths? No one could believe it.

When, in a conquerer's gesture of goodwill, the United States in 1901 introduced polished rice to replace the unrefined rice served in Philippine prisons, the incidence of beriberi rose dramatically. In 1900 there was virtually no beriberi in the prison system. In January 1902 there were 169 cases; in October, there were 579 more. Nothing could stop the spread of beriberi, and the inmates kept dying. After almost 5,000 people had contracted the disease in ten months, whole rice was reintroduced to the prisons in a desperate attempt to stop it. By the following February beriberi had been banished.

Eijkman's successor, the Dutch doctor Gerrit Grijns, had by this time reached the conclusion that there was in rice polishings a "protective substance" that was essential for health.

Another doctor, W. L. Braddon, studied different population groups in Malaya and found that those that ate polished rice were subject to beriberi, while those that ate only slightly refined rice were not. Braddon said toxins in the white rice were responsible for the disease. Rice was accepted as the culprit, though the toxin theory was wrong.

Casimir Funk finally proved that there were no toxins in polished rice and set out in 1910 to find the nutritional substance present in unpolished rice that was missing from white rice—the *vitamine*.

It was 10 years later that the scientists Jansen and Donath finally isolated the beriberi-fighting substance in the husks, which was later identified as thiamine.

20 POUNDS OF ONIONS A WEEK

Zoe had heard of the scurvy that made men's breath foul enough to stop a bird in flight, but he was young and believed he could survive anything. Zoe signed on the ship in London.

His gums began to bleed after he had existed for three months on a

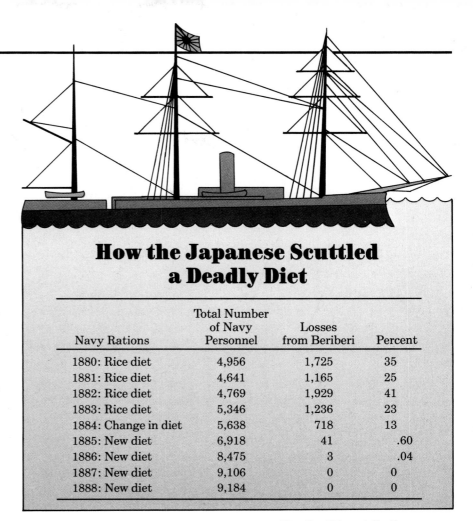

How the Japanese Scuttled a Deadly Diet

Navy Rations	Total Number of Navy Personnel	Losses from Beriberi	Percent
1880: Rice diet	4,956	1,725	35
1881: Rice diet	4,641	1,165	25
1882: Rice diet	4,769	1,929	41
1883: Rice diet	5,346	1,236	23
1884: Change in diet	5,638	718	13
1885: New diet	6,918	41	.60
1886: New diet	8,475	3	.04
1887: New diet	9,106	0	0
1888: New diet	9,184	0	0

diet of biscuits, salted meats and dried beans. He found unwanted jewels on his pillow some mornings. They were his teeth.

It was common at the time to let scurvied men pitch around on deck until they either smashed their heads or fell into the sea. Life wasn't very important in the 18th century, when hundreds of sailors died on each voyage. But this time the captain took pity on Zoe and set him ashore. He crawled up the beach, hungry, stuffing fresh, young grass into his bloody, toothless mouth. Within a few days he had the strength to walk, and soon he felt cured. Another ship picked him up and his story of how *food* reversed the scurvy was spread, finally spawning a cure.

Most plants and most animals are able to build and store vitamin C (ascorbic acid) in their bodies. Man cannot. And it is a lack of dietary vitamin C that causes scurvy.

Millions of city dwellers, besieged soldiers, sailors and prisoners have died over the years from this lack. Many deaths could have been pre-

"Beribieri" is not the Japanese word for "naval battle"—it's a vitamin deficiency disease that once killed over 1,000 Japanese sailors yearly (and put 75 percent of them in sick bay). But then the Japanese conducted an experiment: they sent 2 ships on long voyages, the crew of one eating their traditional white rice rations, the crew of the other eating oatmeal, vegetables, fish, meat and condensed milk (the same diet eaten by British sailors, who were free of beriberi). When the boats returned months later, more than two-thirds of the crew on the white rice ship had beriberi. Only 14 men on the other ship had the disease—and they had refused the British-type rations and eaten white rice. After that, *all* Japanese sailors ate the new diet, and beriberi—caused by a steady fare of thiamine-poor white rice—was scuttled.

vented. As with beriberi, the common sense of a few was ignored for years by the educated and powerful.

A Dutch physician recommended oranges to sailors for scurvy in 1564. In 1639, John Woodall was the first English physician to prescribe citrus fruits, particularly lemons, for the treatment of scurvy. James Lind, a British naval surgeon and the conquerer of scurvy, repeated the advice over a century later after being prompted to conduct research by the story of Zoe. The British navy waited almost another 50 years before giving in to this wisdom.

It had been over 200 years since the Dutch physician spoke—200 years of misery for sailors, whose lives fueled the age of exploration that began at the end of the 15th century with voyages such as Vasco da Gama's trip around the Cape of Good Hope. During this voyage, 100 out of 160 men had to be thrown overboard, their bodies rotted by scurvy.

Exploration continued with voyages such as that of Jacques Cartier. Over 90 percent of his crew was disabled by swollen, blackened legs. Indians saved them by brewing tea made from the vitamin C-rich bark and leaves of a tree, now believed to have been white cedar.

Despite the success of the bark and the use of fruits and vegetables by other sea captains—including James Cook, whose crews were remarkably healthy because they were forced under threat of a lashing to eat a diet that sometimes included 20 pounds of onions a week— little progress was made in scurvy prevention. Sea captains were still losing so many men it is a wonder that some of the ships returned.

The lack of progress was due to medicine's hesitancy to ascribe disease to nutrition, a lack of knowledge of vitamins and the fact that scurvy was often confused with other diseases, especially venereal disease.

Finally, in 1795, one year after Lind's death, two surgeons convinced the British navy to try lemons. Scurvy ceased to exist on royal navy ships. However, crews on some merchant ships were given less expensive, less effective limes, a practice that resulted in several cases of scurvy and was the source of the

well-known nickname for British sailors—"limeys."

Although scientists knew there was an antiscurvy factor in lemons, many failed at attempts to separate the pure vitamin from lemon juice. But vitamin C was finally found, by accident, in 1928 by Albert Szent-Györgyi. Szent-Györgyi once said, "Vitamins . . . will help us to reduce human suffering to an extent which the most fantastic mind would fail to imagine."

BOTTLING THE SUN SO CHILDREN CAN SHINE

Rickets was a scourge from medieval times through the dark days of the Industrial Revolution and well into the 20th century. Because it rarely

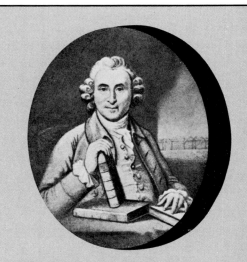

The End of Scurvy

James Lind, a surgeon in the British navy during the 18th century, proved that scurvy was a deficiency disease caused by a lack of certain foods (later found to be those rich in vitamin C). Here's his account of the experiment that supplied the proof.

"On the 20th May, 1747, I treated twelve patients who had scurvy.

resulted in death, it was allowed to fester among populations. And people—especially children—with curved spines, bent legs and swollen joints began to seem normal. There were too many other opportunities for horrible death to worry about a condition that just made one miserable. The disease is caused by a lack of vitamin D, and could have been cured by pleasant days in the sun or unpleasant spoonfuls of cod-liver oil. Unfortunately for children living in cities, especially in England during the Industrial Revolution, work hours were so long that the children were rarely outside during the day, and the skies were so full of coal dust and smoke that the sun's rays rarely made it to the cobblestone streets. And though it was known that Scottish fishermen had prevented

rickets for years with cod-liver oil, most doctors ignored the cure for many years.

One of the earliest sensible theories concerning rickets was proposed by Francis Glisson in the mid-17th century. He concluded that a bad environment caused rickets. Glisson didn't consider diet as a cause, but his observation led to the realization that a lack of sun was a factor. The environmental factor was cited by numerous researchers over the next 150 years, but nothing concrete was established and rickets continued to deform people, especially in England.

Cod-liver oil, the bane of youthful taste buds, was widely used to treat rickets in the 19th century due to the work of several physicians, most notably Armand Trousseau. He treated his patients with cod-liver and other fish-liver oils, sunshine and butter, proving—to himself at least—that diet and sunshine played a vital role in rickets. His findings, along with so many wise deductions of the day, were largely lost in the quest for a rickets-causing germ.

Fortunately, by the early 20th century two separate (but in the end complementary) theories developed. One held that rickets was due to environmental factors, especially a lack of sun, the other that diet was involved. Scientists "relearned" Trousseau's theory. Dr. Kurt Huldschinsky, for example, placed deformed, listless children from Berlin under mercury quartz lamps (which duplicate the sun's ultraviolet rays) and their limbs straightened after two months.

At the same time, in England, Edward Mellanby proved the old wives' tale about using cod-liver oil to cure rickets was actually a scientific fact. Researchers across the Atlantic at Johns Hopkins University then presented evidence that cod-liver oil contained at least one vitaminlike substance in addition to vitamin A when E. V. McCollum destroyed the vitamin A with heat and the oil still cured rickets.

No one could reconcile the internal (nutrition) and external (sunlight) aspects of the disease until Alfred Hess of New York discovered that rats whose food had previously

They all had putrid gums, the spots and lassitude, with weakness of their legs. Two of these were ordered each a quart of cider a day. Two others took twenty-five gutts of *elixir vitriol* three times a day. Two others took two spoonfuls of vinegar three times a day. Two patients were put under a course of sea water. Two others had each two oranges and one lemon given them every day. The two remaining patients took the bigness of a nutmeg three times a day.

"The consequence was, that the most sudden and visible good effects were perceived from the use of oranges and lemons; one of those who had taken them, being fit for duty at the end of six days."

Just as scientists have developed technology to reveal the nutritional role of microminerals in our bodies, they have found ways to monitor the minerals lying beneath the earth's surface.

Here's an "X ray" of a hill. The multispectral image was taken by satellite. The colors represent land at different temperatures and reflections of sunlight. Geologists interpret the colors to read the earth like a book.

In this radar portrait of the San Rafael Swell in Utah, scientists read "brown" as sandstone. "Blue' is the sign for shale. As for that large tract colored a glittering copper, it's just sand dunes.

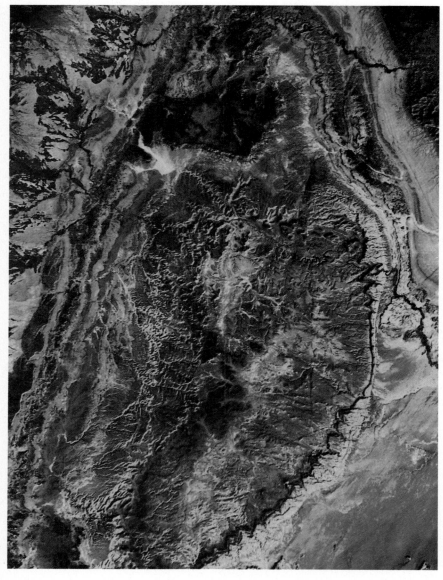

been exposed to the sun did not develop rickets. Fatlike substances in the food were being activated by the ultraviolet rays to produce vitamin D. Today we know that sunlight triggers the body's own production of vitamin D.

Vitamin D was later synthesized, ending up in the vitamin D milk that is now one of the main dietary preventives of rickets.

WHY MINERALS ROCKED THE SCIENTIFIC COMMUNITY

It is not so difficult to understand that the human body needs the vitamins found in certain delicious foods, but who needs to eat rocks

and dirt? Isn't that where minerals come from?

Yes and—thankfully—no.

Minerals are also found in water, meat, vegetables and fruits. But, until recently, modern man didn't think too much about minerals; tin was for cans and cans were for goats. Fortunately, the remarkable relationship between minerals and health has surfaced during this century, when most dietary mineral discoveries were made. Nutritionists now say that tin may be essential for good health. So might vanadium, nickel, silicon and a host of other minerals. Yet these substances still remain something of a mystery. The government has set few Recommended Dietary Allowances (RDAs) for minerals and scientists debate over what the best mineral levels are for humans. (Some minerals can be toxic if taken in large enough doses.)

Zinc, however, has been one of the most widely studied minerals. It has been shown to prevent sexual and physical dwarfism and to help cure a number of serious skin problems. Yet all this is very recent, as far as science is concerned. In 1869, a scientist deduced that zinc was necessary for the growth of mold. That's not the most exciting discovery in history—except perhaps for the mold—but it led eventually to a search for zinc in humans, where it was found in the liver.

Zinc was left on the wayside as just another substance among many in living animals until 1934, when it was proved essential for the growth of healthy mice. As a result, scientists began to study the effects of zinc on humans. In 1944 it was determined that zinc was essential for the elimination of carbon dioxide, a poisonous by-product of metabolism. It was later shown that zinc has a lot to do with the way we look and how we develop sexually.

One of the main researchers into zinc was Ananda S. Prasad, M.D., Ph.D., who must have looked at his experimental subjects with a mixture of awe and disgust. These young Iranian and Egyptian men were oddly stunted and had no facial or pubic hair. They were what scientists call "hypogonadal [sexual] dwarves." And as if that problem wasn't enough, they had rough skin and suffered from enlarged livers and spleens.

Dr. Prasad examined their diet. It consisted of bread, beans, a little white cheese and, very rarely, meat. He thought back to experiments with animals in the lab where sexual dwarfism was induced with a zinc-deficient diet and realized that the men were probably low on zinc. And when he tested the blood levels of the Egyptians for the mineral, he found they *were* deficient. When later researchers supplemented the diets of sexual dwarves with very small amounts of zinc, the men emerged from their arrested puberty.

These zinc studies had many ramifications, the most important of which was to illustrate that some minerals are needed in only "trace" amounts—but that they're no less important than the so-called major minerals like calcium, phosphorus, potassium and magnesium.

A more unusual trace mineral is selenium, first discovered in 1818 by the Swedish scientist Jöns Jacob Berzelius. The mineral has a mixed ancestry. It was first seen as a killer, but is now praised as a lifesaver with possible beneficial effects on cancer.

Berzelius discovered selenium when he scraped the mineral out of sulfuric acid vats in a factory. After identifying it, he left off further research on the mineral, and selenium wasn't studied intensely again until it was implicated in the 1930s for two devastating diseases that struck animals on selenium-rich soil. The mineral's image as a toxin continued until 1957, when a researcher discovered that *small* amounts of selenium were essential to the *health* of animals. Later, the U.S. Food and Drug Administration (FDA) approved it as a feed additive, and farmers and ranchers have used it to prevent a variety of veterinary illnesses.

Human beings haven't been quite as fortunate. Only in the past few years has selenium been recognized as a disease fighter in man. Now scientists believe that selenium may fight cancer by serving as a shield against cancer-causing substances (carcinogens) that enter our bodies every day. Chemistry profes-

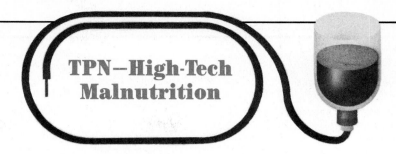

TPN—High-Tech Malnutrition

TPN is total parenteral nutrition—the feeding by tube of a patient who can't eat. And a problem with it has alerted doctors to one of their nutritional blind spots—our need for trace minerals.

"Evidence of metal deficiencies has rarely been seen in man, but the increasing use of total parenteral nutrition . . . has produced a crop of reports of deficiencies of trace elements," says a report in the *British Medical Journal.* It turns out that medical technologists didn't think that some of the newly discovered trace elements were important enough to include in TPN solutions—but they found out differently. And did something about it. A "Statement by an Expert Panel" in the *Journal of the American Medical Association* said that "this undesirable situation requires remedial action" and recommended that zinc, copper, chromium and manganese "be made available" in TPN solutions.

sor Gerhard Schrauzer, Ph.D., believes the mineral slows cell division long enough for carcinogen-damaged cells to repair their chromosomes. He believes that an adequate supply of selenium could help prevent many types of cancer, including breast, lung and skin cancer.

While no minimum daily requirement has been set, scientists all over the world are looking into the benefits of the mineral. While it took over 150 years to take selenium from the blacklist and put it in the "essential" category, perhaps this long-delayed awakening will push scientists to investigate other trace minerals in our bodies and see just how important they are.

2

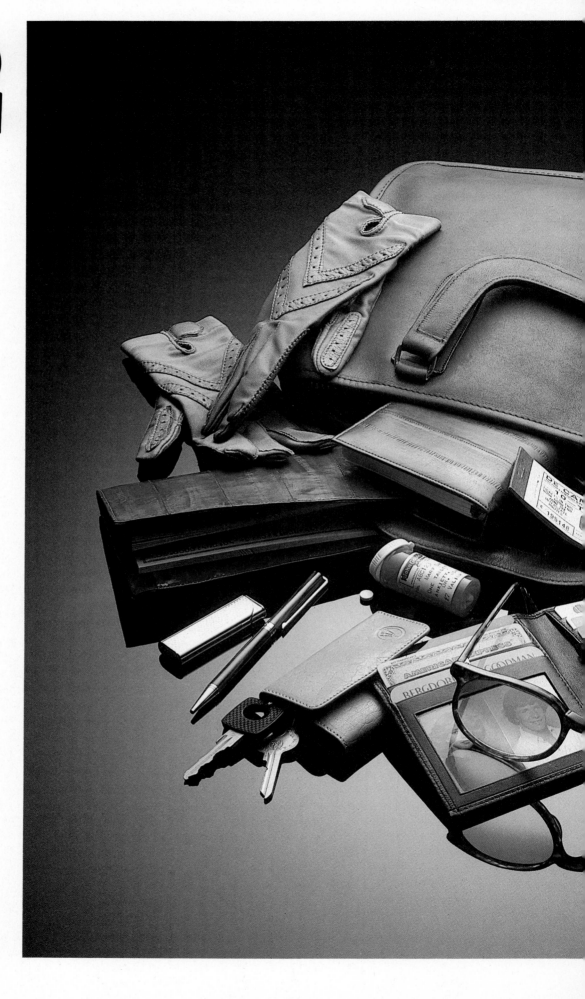

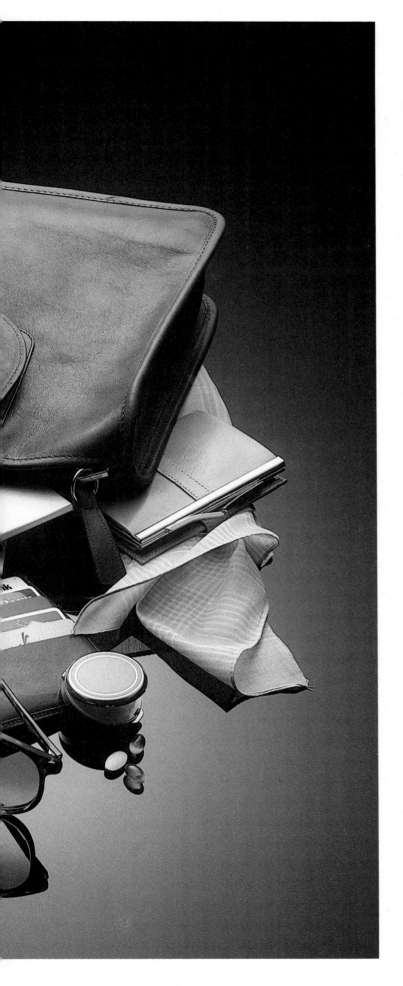

Why You Need Food Supplements

Factory food, pollution, stress—they all drain you of nutrients. Here's how to plug the leak.

Ask your doctor if you need vitamin or mineral supplements, and most likely he'll tell you that you get all the nutrients you need from food. "Healthy people don't need supplements as long as they eat a balanced diet," is the standard reply.

Yet millions of people take vitamin and mineral supplements every day. In fact, a survey of the patients of ten doctors showed that nearly two-thirds of those patients took supplements without the physicians' say-so, and 80 percent thought they had more energy as a result. Were they deluding themselves? Or were the supplements really making them feel better?

The answer to the second question is probably yes. Most doctors categorically state that practically no one besides pregnant women, nursing mothers and people with extremely unusual diets—like strict vegetarians or anorexics—need supplements. Yet when pressed to reconsider, they will concede that people who overindulge in coffee, cigarettes or alcohol burn up or flush out large amounts of vitamins and minerals. And it's a well-known fact that people taking prescription drugs can suffer drug-induced nutrient deficits. Doctors are fully aware, for example, that women taking oral contraceptives run a high risk of vitamin B_6 (pyridoxine) deficiency. New scientific evidence also has shown that stress and pollution—standard ingredients in the pressure cooker of modern life—increase our need for many nutrients. Add to that the reams of research showing that people with frequent colds, skin problems, indigestion, inflamed gums and other annoying health problems often get better when their diets are beefed up with supplements, and almost everyone falls into one or more of the categories of people who need supplements.

But if people really do need extra nutrition, why do government scientists—the supposed experts who put together the Recommended Dietary Allowances—set those vitamin-level guidelines so low you can just about satisfy them with a hepped-up bowl of cereal?

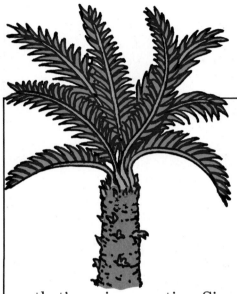

Going Native? Take Calcium Supplements

Nutritional supplements seem like a recent invention, a modern way to squeeze the essence out of a food and bottle it. But that's a misconception. Since ancient times— and in primitive societies today—native peoples have always eaten concentrated or special foods that supply high levels of a particular nutrient. Take calcium, for instance.

In New Guinea, villagers burn the leaves of the sago palm (pictured above), collect the calcium-rich ash and eat it.

In certain African villages, pregnant and nursing women eat edible, calcium-rich clay eggs fashioned by fellow villagers.

And in the highlands of Peru, Indians consume "supplements" known as *cal* and *llipta*. To make *cal*, they burn and grind calcium-containing rocks and add the powder to porridge. To make *llipta*, they burn grain stalks and mix the ash with water to form a paste that is dried in the sun to form cakes. Between these foods, the Peruvians glean an average of about 1,100 milligrams of calcium over and above their regular diet. Oddly enough—or perhaps not so oddly—that's the amount of calcium that some U.S. doctors now suggest is a must for women. To reach that level, they don't recommend eating *llipta*, of course— just taking calcium supplements.

AN "ALLOWANCE" THAT WON'T PAY THE BILLS

The RDAs are the daily amounts of various essential vitamins and minerals that, in the opinion of the government's Food and Nutrition Board of the National Academy of Sciences, are "estimated to exceed the [nutritional] requirements of most individuals."

What that really means is that the RDAs are intended to minimize the risk of severe, disease-causing nutritional deficiencies—*and nothing more.* In no way do they ensure optimum health.

"The RDAs are not designed to cover nutritional needs that may be elevated as the result of disease, stress or the chronic use of certain drugs," says Alfred E. Harper, Ph.D., professor of nutritional sciences and biochemistry at the University of Wisconsin in Madison. "Such conditions require specific individual attention. Also, RDAs do not take into account losses of nutrients that occur during food storage and preparation."

Others are even more critical of the RDAs.

"Everyone has *individualized* nutritional needs," says H. Curtis Wood, Jr., M.D., a nutrition-oriented physician from Philadelphia. "And a person may also vary rather widely in his requirements from day to day, depending on stress, exercise, diet and so on. There are so many things that can act as antagonists [nutrient destroyers]. It's just unrealistic to think that the RDAs will give you all the nutrients you need."

Yet, suppose for a moment that the RDAs were ample—could you really get RDA levels of vitamins and minerals from that "balanced diet" your doctor talks about?

A DIET THAT'S OFF-BALANCE

Probably not. A "balanced diet" to most people means the "four food groups" we all learn about in elementary school: milk and milk products, meats, fruits and vegetables and cereals. Using those criteria, a hot dog on a white bun with pickle relish and a dessert of apple pie and ice cream would qualify as a "balanced" meal. But it has little to offer in the way of vitamins and minerals. As a matter of fact, analysis of the diets of 212 college students who selected their meals from the four food groups showed that a full two-thirds of them came up short of the RDA for vitamin E, vitamin B_6, iron and zinc. And only two-thirds met the RDA for folate (a B vitamin) and magnesium.

And in a separate study of the dietary habits of college women at Cornell University, dietitians and researchers concluded, "It is apparent that, for most young women, the only feasible way to reach the [RDA] for iron is to use an iron supplement."

But college students aren't the only people who have poor eating habits. We all come up short. Since

Even "Wasted" Vitamins Help Protect Us

"I can't understand what good it does to take all those high-priced vitamins and minerals," say skeptics. "All they do is go right through you. The only thing you get from taking more than you need is the most expensive urine in town."

That type of argument is a source of confusion to people who *know* they feel better after taking vitamin supplements. And it raises serious doubts, too: "Am I really popping a bunch of unnecessary pills—and wasting a lot of money, to boot?"

Alan Gaby, M.D., who emphasizes nutrition and preventive medicine in his practice in Baltimore, Maryland, explained how even "wasted" vitamins help protect us.

"When you take a nutritional supplement, some part of it ends up in your urine and is excreted, but that isn't bad. There are at least 2 ways a nutrient can be beneficial to the body even though it eventually gets excreted: Its presence in the urine may promote good health in the bladder and kidneys, and the nutrient may perform a useful function somewhere else in the body before it's excreted."

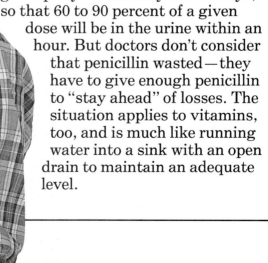

So the skeptics are wrong to believe that any excreted nutrients are excesses the body doesn't need. The process, explains Dr. Gaby, works much like penicillin therapy for various infections. The goal of penicillin therapy is to keep an effective level in the blood and tissues at all times. The larger and more frequent the dose, the more penicillin will be on hand at any one time. On the other hand, the drug is rapidly excreted by the kidneys, so that 60 to 90 percent of a given dose will be in the urine within an hour. But doctors don't consider that penicillin wasted—they have to give enough penicillin to "stay ahead" of losses. The situation applies to vitamins, too, and is much like running water into a sink with an open drain to maintain an adequate level.

the early 1900s (when nutritional data gathering first started), eating habits have changed as drastically as fashions in clothing. And our new diets are somewhat threadbare.

"Consumers [have] moved from . . . bulky, complex carbohydrates (whole grains, tubers, fruits, vegetables) and unprocessed fresh foods, to the consumption of large amounts of animal proteins and fats [and] highly refined flour, sugar and processed foods of all kinds," says Ruth B. Weg, Ph.D., of the Ethel Percy Andrus Gerontology Center at the University of Southern California in Los Angeles.

That's the big picture. In terms of everyday life, the U.S. Department of Agriculture's (USDA) Nationwide Food Consumption Survey showed that on a typical day, only 7 to 8 percent of the people in this country ate either dark green or yellow vegetables—two primary food sources of vitamins A and C and thiamine. Fewer than one-third of men aged 19 to 50 ate citrus fruits or drank citrus juice. (They might be downing soft drinks instead—the USDA reported that "use of soft drinks" is "considerably greater" than it was in the past. And sugary colas and the like not only deliver little or no nutrition, they also deplete the body of thiamine.) The same study revealed that women, including teenagers, are low in iron and calcium—without a doubt two of the minerals most important to women's health.

Americans' constant battle with

When home economists from the USDA studied the diets of nearly 40,000 Americans, they discovered that at least one-third consumed less than 70 percent of the government's RDAs for calcium, iron, magnesium and vitamin B$_6$. In the case of some nutrients, the people who need the most got the least—middle-aged women, for instance, who must get high levels of calcium to keep their bones from thinning, had a dismal intake. And when you consider that many experts believe the RDAs are set too low, you see why most Americans would probably be healthier if they took nutritional supplements.

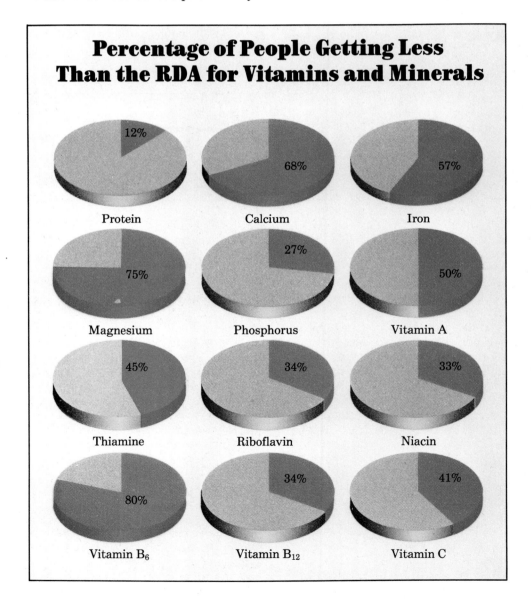

Percentage of People Getting Less Than the RDA for Vitamins and Minerals

12% Protein	68% Calcium	57% Iron
75% Magnesium	27% Phosphorus	50% Vitamin A
45% Thiamine	34% Riboflavin	33% Niacin
80% Vitamin B$_6$	34% Vitamin B$_{12}$	41% Vitamin C

Canning: The Great Vitamin Massacre

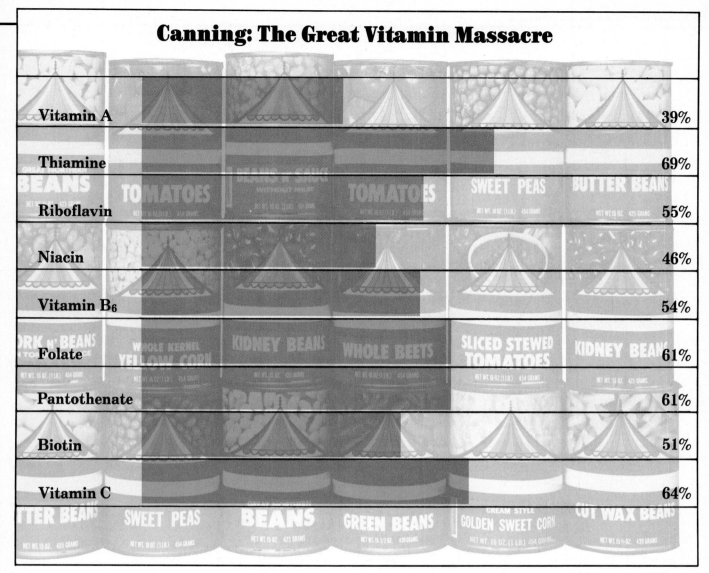

Vitamin A	39%
Thiamine	69%
Riboflavin	55%
Niacin	46%
Vitamin B₆	54%
Folate	61%
Pantothenate	61%
Biotin	51%
Vitamin C	64%

the bulge also produces its share of nutritional casualties. One USDA study showed that about one-third of the people in this country are on a low-calorie diet—and not getting even the RDAs for several vitamins and minerals.

Older people, too, routinely have low-grade deficiencies of calcium, iron, magnesium and vitamins A, C and B complex, according to numerous studies. Those nutritional shortcomings can lower resistance to disease and cause fatigue, headaches, insomnia, irritability and depression—problems that are too often accepted as inevitable features of old age.

THE VITAMIN BANDITS

Aside from the fact that the RDAs are too low and many people have

poor eating habits, a handful of other factors also create the need for vitamin and mineral supplements.

Food Processing and Preparation. A whole, healthy food is a different animal when it's caged in a can, freezer-pack or box. Potatoes, for instance, are *potentially* a regular, reliable source of vitamin C. But today, many people eat potatoes reconstituted from instant mixes, not realizing that these potato products contain no vitamin C whatsoever.

Figures for citrus juice—considered a staple source of vitamin C in the average American diet—are not much better. The simple act of juicing an orange reduces the vitamin C, because this nutrient is very sensitive to oxygen. But orange juice from cardboard cartons has up to 30 percent less vitamin C than fresh-squeezed juice. That wouldn't be so bad, but up to 40 percent of the C

This graph shows that vegetables lose *lots* of vitamins when they're canned. (The percentages are averages of vitamin losses from canned asparagus, beets, carrots, corn, cowpeas, green beans, green peas, lima beans, mushrooms, spinach and tomatoes.) The problem with canning is heat and water, both of which can destroy fragile nutrients. As you can see, thiamine (a must for steady nerves) and vitamin C (for a strong immune system) are the most sensitive to canning, but no vitamin escapes unscathed.

that's left is biologically inactive—of no use whatsoever.

The way food is cooked can also leave it bereft of nutrients. When Mary K. Head, Ph.D., formerly of the department of food science at North Carolina State University in Raleigh, investigated the nutritional content of foods that were being served to students at a cafeteria, she found that the way the food was prepared and served caused considerable nutrient loss. Green beans, for example, contained only one-third as much thiamine as official government food tables said they would—thanks to overcooking.

Government studies also have shown that several key foods may not be providing the nutrients we all thought they did. Pork loin is a good example. For years nutritionists believed that a 6-ounce serving of pork loin delivered 5.4 milligrams of iron—a substantial amount. But the USDA has discovered that pork contains only 1.62 milligrams—70 percent less than was previously thought. And beef, the most popular meat in the United States, has 20 percent less iron than was previously thought. (No one knows whether the difference is because current methods of calculating iron are more accurate or if animals have changed physically over the years.)

Additives. Food additives are other factors that prevent top-level nutrition. EDTA, a chemical preservative commonly used in canned or commercially processed foods, is a heavy-duty iron blocker. So are phosphates —food additives used in soft drinks, ice cream, candy, beer and baked goods. (And baked goods that have iron added— that are "fortified" with the mineral— won't make up the difference. The iron used has a very low biological availability and is practically useless.)

"Today, there are more than 3,000 chemicals used in the commercial foods we eat," says Dr. Wood. "And in one way or another, many of them can be [vitamin or mineral] antagonists."

But supplements not only replace the nutrients that additives deny us, they can also defend us against harmful chemicals in food.

Vitamin C, for example, is probably nature's most effective defense against nitrosamines, cancer-causing compounds formed from the nitrites and nitrates used to color and preserve cured meats and other processed foods. Research by Steven R. Tannenbaum, Ph.D., professor of toxicology and food chemistry at Massachusetts Institute of Technology, has shown that when people take vitamin C with nitrates, nitrosamine formation is blocked. (Dr. Tannenbaum gave a total of 2,000 milligrams of vitamin C, equivalent to about 4 quarts of orange juice. Clearly, a supplement is more practical.)

Drinking. You don't have to be a career alcoholic with a pickled liver

20th-century living is downright deadly—there are hundreds of new chemicals and pollutants in the environment that human bodies have never had to cope with before—and many of them can cause serious illnesses like cancer. That's why we all could use extra vitamin C. It disarms many of those substances (like the ones on the list below) before they can mug your health.

Vitamin C Handcuffs Pollutants

Pesticides	Several chlorinated hydrocarbon insecticides
	Several organophosphate insecticides
Heavy metals	Arsenic
	Cadmium
	Cobalt
	Cyanide
	Fluoride
	Lead
	Mercury
	Silica
	Tellurium
Selected hydrocarbons used in industry	Benzanthrone
	Benzene
	Chloroform
	Glycerol
	Hydrazine
	Polychlorinated biphenyls (PCBs)
	Vinyl chloride
Gaseous pollutants	Carbon monoxide
	Ozone

Drugs: One More Reason Why We Need Extra Nutrients

Therapeutic Class	Major Drugs	Nutritional Effect
Anticonvulsants and sedatives	Diphenylhydantoin	Accelerated vitamin D metabolism
	Phenobarbital	Accelerated vitamin K metabolism
	Glutethimide	Folic acid deficiency
		Vitamin B_6 deficiency
Corticosteroids	Cortisone	Accelerated vitamin D metabolism
	Prednisone	Increased vitamin C excretion
		Increased vitamin B_6 requirement
		Increased zinc excretion
		Increased potassium excretion
Alcohol		Thiamine deficiency
		Impaired vitamin B_6 activation
		Folate deficiency
		Increased magnesium excretion
Nonabsorbed antibiotics	Kanamycin	Reduced lactase levels
	Neomycin	Reduced lactase levels
Antitubercular drugs	Isoniazid	Vitamin B_6 deficiency
		Niacin deficiency
Diuretics	Chlorthiazide	Increased potassium excretion
		Increased magnesium excretion
	Spironolactone	Reduced potassium excretion
Hypotensives	Hydralazine	Vitamin B_6 depletion
Anti-inflammatory drugs	Aspirin	Iron depletion
	Indomethacin	Iron depletion
	Phenylbutazone	Folate deficiency
Oral contraceptives and estrogens	Mestranol	Vitamin B_6 deficiency
	Ethinyl estradiol	Vitamin B_6 deficiency
	Conjugated estrogens	Folate deficiency

Taking drugs of any kind is always a trade-off. For every benefit, there are one or more drawbacks. For instance, many drugs create vitamin or mineral deficiencies by blocking nutrient absorption, speeding excretion or otherwise interfering with metabolism. Supplements, however, may make up for nutrient losses.

to suffer alcohol-induced malnutrition. A researcher at Ohio State University reported that six or seven drinks a day for as little as two weeks can throw the digestive system into reverse, causing the small intestine to secrete fluids that flush food from the body before nutrients can be extracted. In other cases, nutrients are simply destroyed or their metabolism is otherwise disturbed. While thiamine, zinc and magnesium are the three nutrients most easily lost by drinking, vitamins A, B_6, B_{12}, C and D, plus folate, riboflavin (vitamin B_2) and calcium also tend to be depleted quickly. In fact, few, if any, nutrients are unscathed by alcohol consumption.

No one knows exactly how much or how often you have to drink before nutrient losses begin to take their toll, but chances are you should use supplements if you're drinking more than one or two glasses of beer, wine or liquor a day.

Smoking. Every cigarette drains the body of 25 milligrams of vitamin C. So even if a smoker is consuming the RDA for vitamin C—60 milligrams a day—it's all for naught. Some researchers maintain that smokers need *at least* 140 milligrams of vitamin C a day to make up for smoke-fostered losses of that nutrient.

Exercise. You are losing a lot more than weight by indulging in regular vigorous physical activity, whether it's jogging or something else. According to research by Daphne A. Roe, M.D., professor of nutrition at Cornell University, exercise increases your need for riboflavin.

In a recent study, Dr. Roe and her colleagues looked at the exercise and eating habits of a group of "normal" young women, aged 21 to 32, over a period of 12 weeks. During the first 6 weeks of the study, the women did not exercise. Then, for the following 6 weeks, they jogged around a track for 30 to 50 minutes each day. At the end of the study, blood tests revealed that the women needed "significantly" higher amounts of riboflavin during the weeks that they were exercising.

What's more, women who lost weight as a result of the exercise program needed more than double the RDA for riboflavin, which is about 1.2 milligrams for women and 1.6 milligrams for men. Dr. Roe noted, however, that even if the women ate more in order to maintain their weights during the exercise program, they still needed "almost double" the RDA for riboflavin.

But replacing the vitamins lost during exercise isn't the only reason an active person needs extra nutrients. Those vitamins can actually make your fitness program *easier* by giving you more strength and endurance.

So says John H. Richardson, M.D., a biology professor at Old Dominion University in Norfolk, Virginia. Dr. Richardson, partly as a doctor and partly as an avid jogger, became interested in the relationship between different nutrients and stamina. So he set up a series of experiments to test the effects of vitamins and minerals on the endurance of lab animals. One of the vitamins was B_6.

Stress Steals Your Nutrition

One doctor claims that a single fit of rage could burn up to 3 grams of vitamin C. That might be a good estimate. Anger—and every other kind of stress—taxes the adrenal glands and robs the body of vitamin C. In fact, the highest concentration of vitamin C in the body is found in the adrenal glands, where its presence—or absence—really counts. But that's not all.

"Stress causes a skyrocketing of nutritional needs," says Arthur C. Hochberg, Ph.D., a nutrition-oriented psychologist in Bala Cynwyd, Pennsylvania. One of the B vitamins in particular, pantothenate, "is withdrawn from the body at an alarming rate and must be replenished," Dr. Hochberg asserts. Also, "during stress there is an increased withdrawal of minerals from the system," he says.

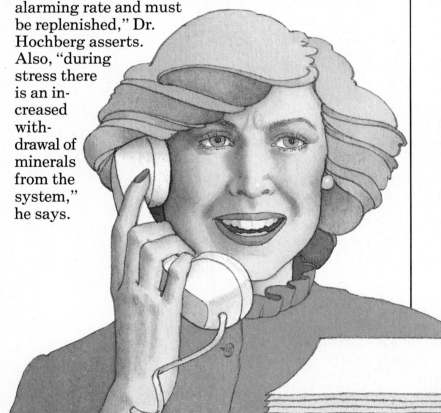

Dr. Richardson assembled two groups of 20 rats. He fed all of them a normal rat chow and conditioned them on an exercise wheel for 30 days. One group was supplemented with B_6 and the other wasn't. At the end of one month, he attached the rats' calf muscles to a spring and measured how many seconds they could maintain a contraction. In human terms, he reported, it was like timing how long you could hold yourself in the "up" position of a chin-up.

The supplemented rats were stronger. "Time to fatigue was measured for all animals," he wrote in the *Journal of Sports Medicine and Fitness*. "Results indicate that contraction time for B_6 animals was significantly longer than [for] controls. This study suggests that vitamin B_6 increases stamina."

Dr. Richardson believes B_6 will work for people as well as animals. "In terms of performance or well-being," he said, "I think we could function on a higher level if we took this nutrient."

Pollution. Supplements help protect you against pollution. Lead absorption, for example, is blocked in the gastrointestinal tract by nutrients like calcium and iron. Adequate riboflavin and niacin help shield you against pesticides. And vitamin E can protect the lungs from damage caused by ozone, the highly toxic pollutant gas that's a major ingredient in smog. Vitamin C protects against cadmium toxicity in animals. (Cadmium can raise blood pressure.) Vitamin C also modifies the dangers of arsenic, cyanide, lead, mercury, benzene, vinyl chloride, carbon monoxide, PCBs and several insecticides. All told, vitamin C has been reported to interact with over 50 chemical pollutants.

Vitamin E doesn't only stop ozone. A group of researchers at the University of Maryland in College Park fed laboratory animals varying amounts of vitamin E and lead. The animals with the lowest intake of vitamin E accumulated the most lead—a good indication that vitamin E blocks lead absorption. And lead is one of the worst heavy metal pollu-

tants because of its presence in auto exhaust.

Vitamin A, too, strengthens our nutritional armor. Scientists at the National Cancer Institute found that rats fed a diet deficient in vitamin A had an increased uptake of toxic chemicals. As with vitamins C and E, diet alone may not provide protective amounts of this nutrient.

And *everyone* needs protection against pollution, no matter where they live.

"Air pollution is not confined to metropolitan areas," says Daniel Menzel, Ph.D., a researcher at Duke University Medical Center in Durham, North Carolina. "Rain made highly acidic by air pollution is a uniform phenomenon east of the Rocky Mountains. The amount of ozone in certain rural areas of New Jersey is greater than in downtown Manhattan."

Dr. Menzel says that the amount of vitamin E in the typical American diet—9 international units (I.U.)—is probably too low to maintain good health, let alone shield a person from the stress of air pollution. To protect his own health, Dr. Menzel takes 200 I.U. of vitamin E every day.

"The concept of the RDA should be broadened to take into account the effects of ubiquitous pollutants on human health," says Edward J. Calabrese, Ph.D., professor of environmental health at the University of Massachusetts in Amherst.

And with all this evidence, your personal concept of your nutritional needs should probably be broadened, too—to include supplements.

3

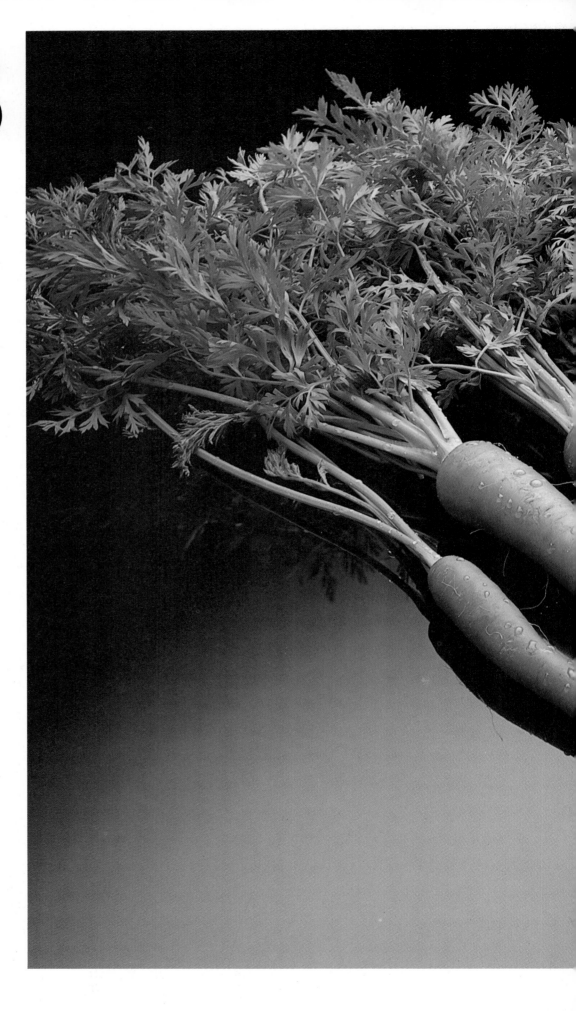

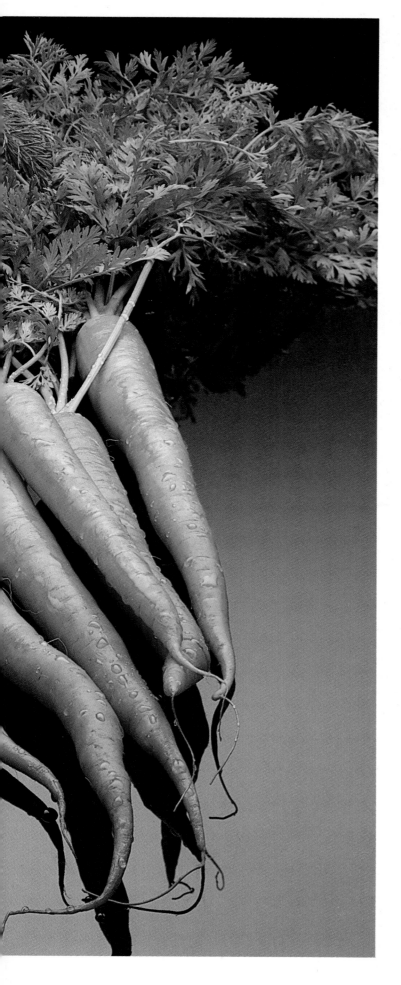

Vitamin A— From A to Z

It seems hard to believe that one nutrient works in so many ways to guard health, but nature is rather adept at such miracles.

I t's only fitting that vitamin A should come first alphabetically in the long list of necessary nutrients discovered by science, because no other vitamin or mineral is more basic to good health.

Vitamin A is the foremost example of the awesome versatility nature has packed into vitamins. Unlike drugs, which do just a few specialized things, vitamin A helps to regulate and maintain a whole range of essential functions inside our bodies.

For example, vitamin A is a key factor in having smooth, healthy-looking skin. It's also vital for sharp vision, especially at night. And, less obviously but just as importantly, this nutrient maintains the moisture in the mucous membranes that line your mouth, respiratory passages and urinary tract—thus ensuring resistance to infection. Vitamin A also bolsters your body's natural immunity, so necessary in safeguarding against infectious diseases and even against cancer. In recent years, even the conservative National Research Council has pronounced that eating foods rich in vitamin A is an important step in lowering the risk of developing certain kinds of cancer.

Vitamin A also helps to counter the damaging effects of stress, as well as to speed wound healing. Moreover, it can detoxify certain chemicals. And multitalented vitamin A does even more.

It's involved in sexual functioning, in that a shortage can lead to female problems related to menstruation and male problems of infertility.

On top of all that, this versatile vitamin may have a profound effect on whether or not we fall prey to heart disease, high blood pressure, stroke and peptic ulcer. That's the conclusion of a major study conducted in Israel by Aviva Palgi, Ph.D., who analyzed 28 years' worth of data in order to determine the cumulative effects of dietary changes on specific mortality rates.

Dr. Palgi, who has conducted research in nutrition at Harvard Medical School and is now at the American Health Foundation in New York City, found that between 1949 and 1977, the Israeli death rate from heart disease more than doubled, while the death rates from high blood pressure, stroke and peptic ulcer also increased significantly. Meanwhile, during that same time span, Israelis had changed their eating habits, so that by 1970 they were consuming more fat and fewer complex carbohydrates. Dr. Palgi not only looked at these obvious dietary factors, she also examined the direct effect of specific vitamins and minerals on the diseases mentioned.

And that's where vitamin A comes in.

"Vitamin A," says Dr. Palgi, "consistently had a significant negative association with mortality rates." This means that the more vitamin A individuals in the study consumed, the less likely they were to suffer from heart disease, high blood pressure, stroke and peptic ulcer.

Dr. Palgi's study, published in the *American Journal of Clinical Nutrition,* concludes by suggesting that if people ate much less fat and at the same time consumed more vitamin A, they might live longer, healthier lives.

"We are just beginning to see the benefits of vitamin A in the diet," Dr. Palgi says, "and it's very exciting.

"Right now we know that 5,000 I.U. of vitamin A daily is an absolute requirement for health. But for people in a predisease state, more may be needed. I know that in view of the results of my study I am more conscious of my diet and I try to eat plenty of vitamin A-rich foods while also keeping my total fat intake as low as possible."

ARE YOU SHORTCHANGING YOURSELF?

For all its importance, you'd think that vitamin A would be generously distributed in many foods. Dark green and yellow vegetables, many fruits, liver, butter and eggs are all good sources of the nutrient. But in spite of nature's generosity, many people still manage to shortchange themselves—day after day.

The amount of vitamin A we consume from fresh and processed fruits and vegetables has dropped in the last 50 years. According to the results of federal dietary surveys, the average American manages to eat just 3,860 I.U. of vitamin A per day from those sources, down from 4,330 I.U. in the 1925-29 period.

When we overlook foods such as carrots, sweet potatoes, broccoli and spinach—all high in vitamin A—or choose a precooked meal instead, we can get into even more nutritional trouble. For example, researchers at Pennsylvania State University found that 99 percent of customers eating meals at fast food outlets were getting *less* than one-fourth of their daily allowance for vitamin A. In fact, the researchers pointed out, "There were no rich sources of vitamin A on the menu of the two restaurants we studied."

Can You Overdose on Vitamin A?

If you see polar bear liver on the menu, don't order it. That meat is so high in vitamin A it's poisonous. But if you don't dine out regularly at the North Pole, vitamin A isn't much of a threat. True, your liver stores unused vitamin A, and if it builds up beyond a certain point you can get sick. But such cases are very rare. For instance, one report told of a 3-year-old girl given 200,000 I.U. of vitamin A a day—an amount that defies common sense. (For adults, the maximum daily dose should be 25,000 I.U.)

And even if you were to take too much, there are lots of early warning signals: deep bone pain, very dry skin, headaches and hair loss. Simply stopping your intake of A will clear up the symptoms. When they're gone, you can take the vitamin again, but at a lower dosage.

Fast food patrons aren't the only ones lacking vitamin A. Older people as a group seem to be at special risk. A Colorado State University study of 70 women uncovered startling evidence of vitamin A deficiency. The women ranged in age from 62 to 99 years; some lived in nursing homes, others in private homes. The investigators found that 21 percent of the women obtained "less than adequate levels" of vitamin A from their food. In this case, "less than adequate" was defined as a mere two-thirds—or less—of the RDA of 4,000 I.U. for women in this age group.

Such deficits are even more alarming when we realize that many people apparently need even more than the government-set RDA for vitamin A to achieve maximum health. A study conducted at the University of Alabama involving 1,056 dentists and their wives found that individuals had fewer symptoms and health complaints as their vitamin A intake went up. The best level of health was reported by those getting approximately 33,000 I.U. of vitamin A daily.

The *Journal of the National Cancer Institute* also published a study of importance. In a nutshell, it said that people who develop lung cancer—which kills more Americans than any other form of cancer—have a history of lower vitamin A intake than people who do not develop lung cancer.

To check that study, Micheline Mathews-Roth, M.D., of Harvard Medical School, and other doctors are testing the effects of beta-carotene on health. Beta-carotene (also called pro-vitamin A) is a natural pigment in vitamin A-rich vegetables and fruits that converts to vitamin A once inside the body. Carrots, sweet potatoes, dark leafy greens, apricots, cantaloupes and winter squash are all sources of beta-carotene.

"The studies to date show that there is something in beta-carotene-rich foods that has an effect on cancer," says Dr. Mathews-Roth.

You don't have to get rabid about rabbit food, though, because Dr. Mathews-Roth points out that the studies showed that "those who benefited from the beta-carotene in

The Best Food Sources of Vitamin A

Food	Portion	Vitamin A (I.U.)
Beef liver	3 oz.	45,390
Sweet potato	1 medium	11,940
Carrots, sliced, cooked	½ cup	8,140
Spinach, cooked	½ cup	7,290
Cantaloupe	¼ medium	4,620
Kale, cooked	½ cup	4,565
Broccoli, cooked	1 stalk	4,500
Squash, winter	½ cup	4,305
Mustard greens, cooked	½ cup	4,060
Apricots, fresh	3 medium	2,890
Watermelon	1 slice	2,510
Endive, raw	1 cup	1,650
Leaf lettuce	1 cup	1,050
Asparagus, cooked	4 spears	540
Peas, fresh, cooked	½ cup	430
Green beans, cooked	½ cup	340
Yellow corn	½ cup	330
Parsley, dried	1 tbsp.	303
Egg, hard-cooked	1 large	260

fighting cancer weren't eating *huge* amounts of vegetables." However, the studies did show "that people aren't even eating the 3 ounces a day or so that they should be getting."

So, the bottom line is that it's a good idea, in fact a *wise* idea, to get your full allowance of vitamin A every day.

If you take vitamin supplements, you'll want to make sure they include vitamin A. How much? The Recommended Dietary Allowance for vitamin A is 5,000 I.U. daily for men; 4,000 I.U. for women. Pregnant women need at least 5,000 I.U. daily; nursing mothers 6,000 I.U.

Many people take something in the neighborhood of 10,000 to 20,000 I.U. But don't let your enthusiasm get out of hand. Unlike vitamin C and the B vitamins, which are water soluble, excesses of vitamin A are not excreted, but are stored in the liver. A big surplus can cause damage there and throughout the body.

If you prefer to get all your vitamin A from the food you eat, look to the excellent sources listed in the table on page 23.

YOUR BEAUTIFUL BIRTHDAY SUIT

Perhaps vitamin A's most visible benefit is the way it helps our body's largest organ, the skin. Not only does this nutrient keep healthy skin looking beautiful, it also works to remedy a number of skin conditions and diseases. In fact, without adequate vitamin A in the diet, even healthy skin becomes dry, rough and flaky. In extreme cases, the scalp becomes inflamed and scaling leads to dandruff. Or leukoplakia can develop—white patches on the lips, gums, tongue or other mucous membranes in the mouth. Such patches have a tendency to become malignant. Also, because vitamin A deficiency affects the functioning of the skin's sebaceous glands, hair may become dry, weak and brittle.

As you can see, vitamin A is vital to skin health—so vital that many doctors prescribe it as a treatment.

"In general, for all my patients over 50 who have skin changes, I routinely suggest 25,000 units of vitamin A per day," notes dermatologist Irwin I. Lubowe, M.D., in his book *The Modern Guide to Skin Care and Beauty.* Combined with vitamin C and a good multivitamin/mineral supplement, vitamin A is needed "for production and maintenance of skin integrity in the aging," he adds.

Another physician who regularly prescribes vitamin A supplements is August Daro, M.D., of Chicago. He began treating skin problems, but discovered the vitamin also is effective against nonmalignant breast tumors (chronic cystic mastitis).

"I began to use vitamin A for sebaceous cysts of the skin," Dr. Daro says. "And I thought that since the breast tissues derive from the skin, maybe the breast tumors will respond to vitamin A, too. I noticed that these women had dry skin. So I gave them vitamin A, and it worked. I've seen cysts of the breast 2 to 3 centimeters [about 1 inch] in diameter disappear with vitamin A.

"I use vitamin A for any cyst that appears on the skin. And unlike a drug, there are no adverse side effects. I've been in practice for a long, long time and I have never seen a case of vitamin A toxicity. However, I have seen thousands of people who had a deficiency of vitamin A."

MORE THAN SKIN DEEP

Acne vulgaris, or common acne, is another skin disorder that seems to respond well to vitamin A, in combination with other therapies. Acne is probably one of the most common diseases of the skin. It usually occurs on the face, with pimples and blackheads being the most obvious

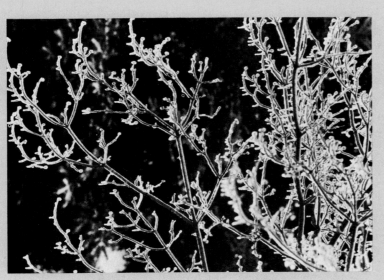

Winterize Your Skin

"Dry skin during winter is a sign of vitamin A depletion," says Carl Reich, M.D., who lives where winter is at its woolliest—Calgary, Alberta. "Vitamin A is a must for the growth of the skin from its basement layer. That layer eventually moves to the surface as skin cells are sloughed off." With adequate vitamin A, he says, "skin lasts longer—it doesn't become scaly and dry and rip off too soon." So protect your skin from the inside out with a diet rich in vitamin A.

symptoms. While acne has been treatable, it has remained incurable.

"Vitamin A has been used by itself to treat acne, but with little success," says Samuel Ayres, Jr., M.D., of Los Angeles. What about combining A and E? He and his colleague, Richard Mihan, M.D., have their acne patients take an average daily dose of 100,000 I.U. of vitamin A and 800 I.U. of vitamin E. "We've had very good results with this treatment," says Dr. Ayres. And the doses of vitamins can usually be reduced after a few months. (These dosages should be taken only under a doctor's supervision.)

The patients also use a topical medication—benzoyl peroxide gel—and are told what foods to avoid. "Extra iodine can aggravate acne, so we advise our patients to avoid iodized salt. Excess milk, fats and sweets also can cause acne to flare up. Many commercial soft drinks contain brominated vegetable oils as stabilizers, which may irritate acne conditions, too. We tell our patients to drink fresh fruit juices."

A synthetic form of vitamin A, 13-cis retinoic acid, is being used to cure very severe acne. ("13-cis" identifies its molecular structure.) One study on 13-cis retinoic acid was done in Leeds, England, where doctors used it to treat eight patients between the ages of 18 and 32. The patients suffered from severe acne—ranging from small pimples to deeply inflamed cysts—that therapy with antibiotics hadn't helped.

The patients took oral 13-cis retinoic acid daily for four months. After one month, the amount of sebum (the skin oil that causes pimples when trapped under the skin by a clogged duct) produced by their sebaceous glands declined by 75 percent. After four months, the patients' acne conditions improved by 80 percent.

A FEAST FOR THE SENSES

Mom was right when she said, "Eat your carrots—they're good for your eyes." But she could have added, "and for your hearing, smell and taste, too." In fact, all the senses

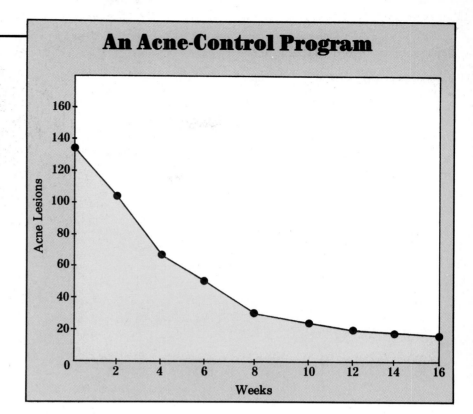

An Acne-Control Program

depend on vitamin A to carry out their jobs. Its role in hearing, for example, has been investigated by Richard A. Chole, M.D., Ph.D., of the University of California at Davis. Dr. Chole, who is associated with that school's department of otorhinolaryngology, has carefully studied what happens to the inner ears of animals that have been deprived of vitamin A.

"We have found," Dr. Chole says, "that most of our vitamin A-deficient animals develop very dramatic *middle* ear changes that I believe lead to a greater incidence of middle ear infections. These changes in the middle ear may very well prove to be more serious than what takes place in the inner ear."

The middle ear is an air-filled cavity that plays a key role in the amplification of sounds.

Vitamin A's importance to the ear doesn't really surprise Dr. Chole. He points out that all the other special senses—vision, smell and taste—have already been shown to depend on the nutrient. In fact, he says, "The receptor cells of all the special senses in mammals are structurally similar" and—with the exception of the hair cells of the inner ear—their dependency on vitamin A for normal function was already a matter of record.

In this experimental trial, 13-cis retinoic acid, a man-made cousin of vitamin A, cured even the most stubborn acne in many cases. Researchers described patients' improvements as "dramatic." It seems that this synthetic form of vitamin A does what vitamin A does—normalizes all the epithelial tissues, including the skin—but does it much more efficiently.

Vitamin A-Rich Recipe: Sweet Carrot Frittata

Makes 2 servings

3 medium carrots, cut into ⅛-inch slices	¾ teaspoon ground cumin
2 teaspoons minced peeled ginger root	½ teaspoon fennel seeds
1 tablespoon butter or margarine	¼ cup chopped walnuts
1 tablespoon honey	4 eggs
¾ teaspoon ground cardamom	1 tablespoon water
	2 teaspoons olive oil

Steam carrots over boiling water for 5 to 7 minutes, until just tender. Set aside and let cool.

Saute ginger in butter or margarine over medium heat for 1 minute. Stir in honey, cardamom, cumin, fennel seeds and nuts. Add carrots. Toss and cook for 3 to 5 minutes, or until glazed. Remove from heat and let cool.

Lightly beat eggs and water and add ¾ of the cooled carrot mixture.

Place a 7- to 8-inch ovenproof skillet over medium-high heat and add olive oil; add eggs when pan is hot. Cook over medium-high heat for 5 to 7 minutes, lifting the sides gently so that uncooked portion flows under cooked portion. Remove from heat and place under broiler, 5 to 6 inches from heat. Broil for 5 to 7 minutes, until top is golden and puffed or until frittata sets firm. Garnish with remaining carrots.

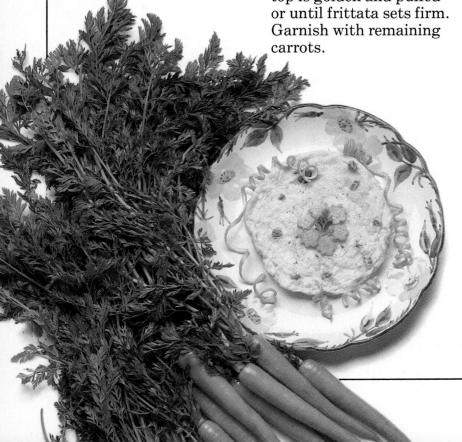

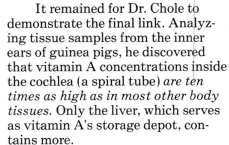

It remained for Dr. Chole to demonstrate the final link. Analyzing tissue samples from the inner ears of guinea pigs, he discovered that vitamin A concentrations inside the cochlea (a spiral tube) *are ten times as high as in most other body tissues.* Only the liver, which serves as vitamin A's storage depot, contains more.

Dr. Chole concluded, "The presence of high concentrations of vitamin A in the inner ear lends credence to the hypothesis that all special sensory receptor cells contain, or are functionally dependent upon, vitamin A."

These findings may help explain the benefical effects of vitamin A supplementation on hearing noted by past researchers. More than a quarter century ago, for example, M. Joseph Lobel, M.D., a New York City physician, reported dramatic improvements in hearing among patients given injections of vitamin A—alone or in conjunction with vitamin B complex.

As Dr. Chole indicates, however, vitamin A's usefulness to the senses is by no means limited to hearing. He cites cases where people regained their sense of smell after taking vitamin A. And researchers at Cornell University have demonstrated that animals deprived of this nutrient lose the ability to differentiate between quinine-flavored, salted and plain water. "These results indicate that vitamin A is required for normal taste function," they note in the journal *Society for Experimental Biology and Medicine.*

THE EYES NEED VITAMIN A

But nowhere is vitamin A's influence on our perceptions more spectacularly evident than in the eyes.

One of the classic signs of vitamin A deficiency is night blindness. That's because in dim light, the remarkable process we call seeing—actually chemical changes turned to electrical impulses turned to mental pictures—requires, at one point, a light-sensitive pigment known as rhodopsin, or visual purple. And the primary source of rhodopsin is vitamin A.

"If the 'lights go out' for a child when dusk approaches, it's quite possible he's suffering from severe vitamin A deficiency . . . ." says Myron A. Winick, M.D., the director of the Columbia University Institute of Human Nutrition. "The primary effect of vitamin A deficiency is damage to the patient's eyes, with problems ranging from night blindness in some cases to irreversible corneal scarring in others."

Heavy drinkers are at special risk for night blindness since alcohol seems to interfere with the liver's ability to store and mobilize vitamin A.

CONTROLLING GLAUCOMA

More serious than night blindness is glaucoma, a condition of increased pressure and fluid buildup inside the eyeball that can lead to total blindness. But here again, there is evidence that vitamin A may have a protective effect.

Dr. Stanley C. Evans, who practices medicine in West Africa, where the incidence of glaucoma is 30 times that in Europe, reported in *Nutritional Metabolism:* "Usually the precipitating cause of many eye disorders, including primary glaucoma, is a vitamin A deficiency." When he gave nutritional supplements, including large doses of A, to a group of patients suffering with restricted vision, blind spots and eye pain, their glaucoma was controlled just as effectively as with conventional drug therapies.

Finally, a prolonged deficiency of vitamin A, coupled with general nutritional deficiencies, leads to xerophthalmia, a condition of abnormal dryness of the eye. Xerophthalmia is the leading cause of blindness in underdeveloped nations. And "although severe manifestations are rare in the United States," says Dr. Winick, "milder effects are frequently encountered, especially among children."

THE BODY'S GUARDIAN

Your body is like a fortress, with "walls" of skin protecting your

Night Vision: How It Works

Night vision depends almost entirely on cylindrical nerve endings in the eye called rods, for they contain a special pigment— rhodopsin, also called visual purple—that helps the eye adapt to changes in light. When light hits the retina (as when high beams of an approaching car stab the eyes), rhodopsin is split into its component parts. Back in the dark again (after the vehicle has passed), normal vision is regained when adequate levels of rhodopsin have been regenerated.

But here's the clincher: Without vitamin A on hand, rhodopsin can't be formed.

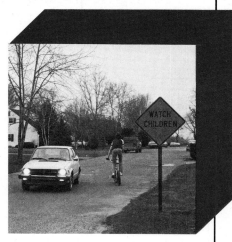
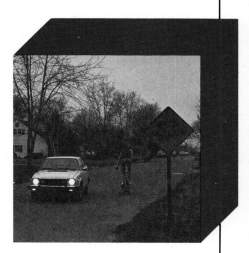

internal organs from attack by sunlight, dust, rain, germs and thousands of potentially deadly invaders.

But no fortress is perfect. Every fortress has gates to allow interaction between the inside and the outside. The body is no exception; it has to eat, breathe, eliminate wastes, hear, see and reproduce. All of these functions require gates to the outside world, and every gate needs a guardian.

Vitamin A is that guardian. Without vitamin A the body quickly loses its ability to keep the invaders at bay.

Consider the respiratory tract. Very little of the air that enters and leaves the lungs each day is so pure that it doesn't contain *something* you'd rather not have in your body. Luckily, the respiratory tract has an efficient mechanism to clean and protect itself. Millions of microscopic

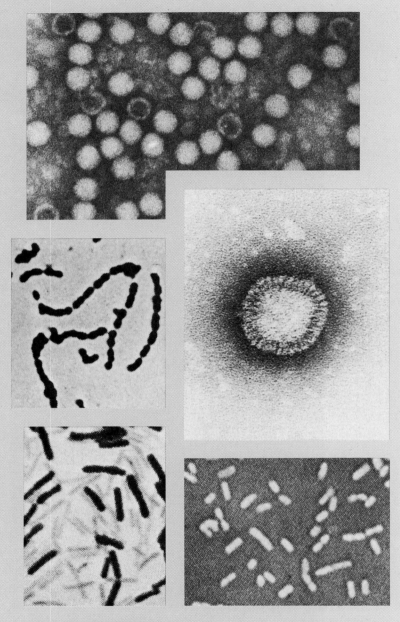

A Mug Shot of the Common Cold (and Accomplices)

The FBI should have *these* tacked up in post offices. At top is a rhinovirus, which causes a *lot* of colds. But the bugs below it—the bacteria streptococcus on the left (responsible for strep throat) and another cold-causing virus on the right—do more than their share of damage. Below them are *B. cereus* on the left and *E. coli* on the right; the latter is a frequent cause of urinary tract infections. All these bad guys have one thing in common: Vitamin A helps control them because it strengthens the mucosa, the lining of the digestive, urinary and respiratory tract where they dig in and start their dirty work.

hairs called cilia line the air passage and sweep a film of mucus outward from the lungs. Dust and other foreign particles are caught by the mucus and carried away.

Even if the air were pure, however, the tremendous volume of it passing over sensitive tissues would quickly dry them out. Constant bathing in mucus keeps these passages moist.

The same is true for the other "gates" of the body. Mucous membranes also guard the mouth, throat, esophagus, digestive system and the genitourinary system. And without adequate vitamin A, these membranes cannot function. Actually, without vitamin A, the body cannot even *produce* mucus-secreting cells. In the case of a deficiency of vitamin A, these membranes not only dry up but are actually *replaced* by hard, horny tissue. That happens in a serious deficiency. In a slight deficiency, the mucous membranes are weakened.

With the gates unguarded, of course, the body is left vulnerable to invasion from foreign elements. Dr. Thomas Moore of Dunn Nutritional Laboratory in Cambridge, England, commenting on his work with rats in *The Vitamins*, says that the most common causes of death among animals deprived of vitamin A are infections of the lining of the respiratory tract, the intestines or the urinary tract.

Inadequate amounts of vitamin A in the body can be the result of more than just not eating right. Any stress—from a feverish cold to a car accident—robs the body of up to 60 percent of its vitamin A. "In such situations," writes Eli Seifter, Ph.D., a nutritional biochemist and a professor at the Albert Einstein College of Medicine in New York City, "large amounts of vitamin A are needed to replace the losses and to stimulate the immunologic responses weakened by the stress."

And one of those "immunologic responses," Dr. Seifter says, is the ability of the mucosa to keep bacteria from inflaming already infected areas.

But vitamin A does more than simply reinforce our barriers against disease, says Dr. Seifter. "The nutrient actually *mobilizes* our infection-fighting white blood cells.

In one of his experiments, Dr. Seifter fed half of his lab animals an adequate amount of vitamin A; the other half was fed ten times that amount. Then they all were exposed to gamma radiation. The highly supplemented animals held up better. "The radiation destroys most but not all of the animals' white blood cells," he says. "The vitamin A stimulates the rate at which the animals regain a normal number of white blood cells, thereby increasing the rate of survival. The highly supplemented animals were able to recoup in a couple of weeks."

In addition, Dr. Seifter has also demonstrated that vitamin A may help fight off the viruses responsible for influenza and the common cold. "We find that vitamin A enhances the immunological response of the body to both types of viruses [DNA and RNA], and this has broad implications," says Dr. Seifter.

SPEEDY RECOVERY FROM SURGERY

Benjamin E. Cohen, M.D., of Houston, Texas, has been studying vitamin A over the years and has found that it boosts the immune response in people who need it most: postsurgical patients.

"It has consistently been found that anesthesia and surgery result in a suppression of the immune response in patients," he says. "Whenever patients are anesthetized, it generally takes a few weeks for their immune response to recover."

Working with colleagues from Australia and England, Dr. Cohen conducted research with patients who were undergoing elective operations. The patients were divided into two groups. One group received vitamin A before, during and after surgery. The other group did not take any vitamin A supplementation.

Dr. Cohen reported his results in the journal *Surgery, Gynecology and Obstetrics*: "By and large, there was a tendency toward a depression of the immune function in patients not taking vitamin A," Dr. Cohen con-cluded. "On the average, patients who *did* take vitamin A did not experience a depression of the immune response at all." Vitamin A seemed to keep the patients' immune defenses functioning normally despite their surgery, giving them a better chance to recover quickly.

AN INVISIBLE GAS MASK

As long as the body's vitamin A supply is adequate, the "gates" do a very efficient job of keeping out invaders. But no gatekeeper is perfect, and the mucous membranes cannot stop *every* foreign particle or substance from entering the body. Chemicals that pollute our air, food and water can make their way into the body.

Aside from living in wet suits and gas masks, there doesn't seem to be much we can do to combat undesirable chemical invaders. Yet

Sinusitis: Nosed Out by Vitamin A

Sinuses are hollow air spaces in the bones of the skull. They are symmetrically arranged in 4 groups of 2. When one of them becomes inflamed (from allergy or infection), sinusitis strikes. The mucous lining swells and pumps out thick mucus. Your ears ring, your head pounds and you can't breathe too well. Enter vitamin A. For vitamin A not only thins mucus, but it is also directly responsible for the production of *healthy* mucus-producing cells. A lack of vitamin A may cause chronic sinusitis, and an extra dose of the nutrient can help clear up a long-standing or new case.

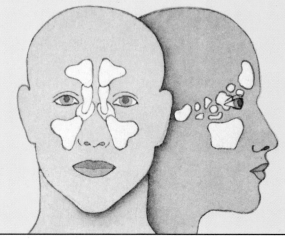

we are not unarmed, according to Dr. Seifter. Research that he and his colleagues have done has led him to believe firmly that vitamin A will help guard against a variety of environmental hazards and stresses.

In a presentation before an American Chemical Society meeting, Dr. Seifter illustrated how the toxicity of a substance is influenced by the nutritional and the general health status of an animal and how those findings relate to humans in the workplace.

In one experiment, Dr. Seifter and his colleagues studied the effects of vitamin A on the toxic compound toluene diamine (TDA). The chemical causes such severe ulceration that the stomach perforates. Death can occur from peritonitis, following a leakage from the stomach.

TDA ingestion causes blood to withdraw from the stomach (humans may identify it as a queasy feeling) and from the skin (similar to the paleness that occurs after a type of stress response). The condition is called ischemia, which means a loss of circulating blood that causes blanching or whitening. Ischemia is an early event leading to stress ulceration and delaying healing of the ulcer.

In animals given only TDA, blanching of the stomach occurred. Animals that received both TDA and vitamin A did not show a blanching effect.

Eventually, the animals on TDA alone developed certain stomach ulcerations, while the animals whose TDA intake was supplemented with vitamin A did not have the stomach ulcerations.

A toxic compound's ability to produce duodenal and stomach ulcers, after a diminished blood supply in those parts of the gastrointestinal tract, can be overcome by vitamin A, Dr. Seifter's research showed.

He says that TDA and some other chemicals either directly or indirectly constrict blood vessels to certain organs like the stomach and skin, while opening up blood vessels elsewhere, especially in muscle. Dr. Seifter and his colleagues speculate that vitamin A prevents that alteration in blood flow pattern from taking place.

A CUSHION AGAINST STRESS

Stress is nothing new. When primitive man met a tiger in the forest, he could either do battle or run as fast as his legs could carry him. What he experienced is called *acute* stress, where the threat is immediate and the response must be instantaneous. If you've ever had a near-accident, you've felt acute stress. But a second kind of stress also exists—a stress that is prolonged and unresolved. Called *chronic* stress, it propels the body into an unnatural level of excitement. One physical result of chronic stress can be enlargement of the adrenal glands. And if the stress is severe enough, bleeding and even tissue death can result.

"Environmental stresses and sicknesses tend to cause the adrenal glands to enlarge and even to hemorrhage," says Dr. Seifter.

But vitamin A can stop that damage, as Dr. Seifter and co-workers Anthony N. Critselis, M.D., and Giuseppe Rittura, Ph.D., discovered. In one of a series of experiments carried out by the trio, rats were given a large dose of a potent cancer-causing chemical, DMBA. Normally, such a dose causes extreme injury to the adrenal glands, resulting in death of glandular tissue. But when animals were fed diets heavily supplemented with vitamin A for three days prior to exposure to DMBA, their adrenals were protected.

The protective effect lies in vitamin A's ability to prevent the adrenal from enlarging. By doing so, vitamin A also blocks a secondary consequence—the shrinkage or shriveling up of the thymus gland. This blocking action is important because when the thymus shrinks, the body's ability to fight disease is crippled.

VITAMIN A FIGHTS POLLUTANTS

These findings may supply the missing pieces in a number of perplexing medical puzzles. For example, researchers at the Hebrew University-Hadassah Medical School in Jerusalem reported that animals exposed to the industrial pollutants

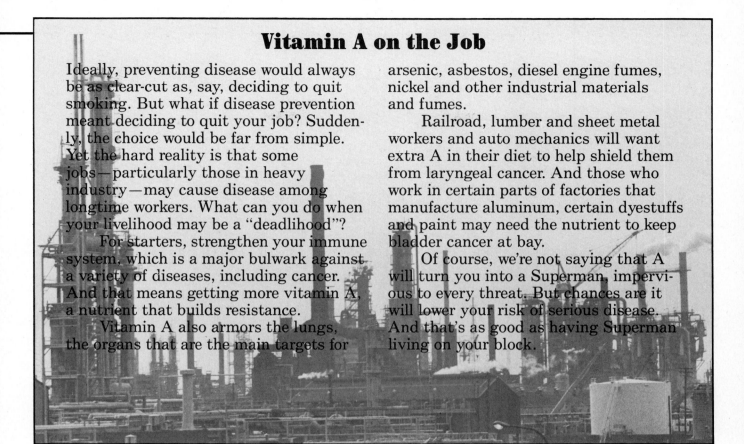

Vitamin A on the Job

Ideally, preventing disease would always be as clear-cut as, say, deciding to quit smoking. But what if disease prevention meant deciding to quit your job? Suddenly, the choice would be far from simple. Yet the hard reality is that some jobs—particularly those in heavy industry—may cause disease among longtime workers. What can you do when your livelihood may be a "deadlihood"?

For starters, strengthen your immune system, which is a major bulwark against a variety of diseases, including cancer. And that means getting more vitamin A, a nutrient that builds resistance.

Vitamin A also armors the lungs, the organs that are the main targets for arsenic, asbestos, diesel engine fumes, nickel and other industrial materials and fumes.

Railroad, lumber and sheet metal workers and auto mechanics will want extra A in their diet to help shield them from laryngeal cancer. And those who work in certain parts of factories that manufacture aluminum, certain dyestuffs and paint may need the nutrient to keep bladder cancer at bay.

Of course, we're not saying that A will turn you into a Superman, impervious to every threat. But chances are it will lower your risk of serious disease. And that's as good as having Superman living on your block.

PCBs showed degenerative changes in the adrenal glands.

PCBs (polychlorinated biphenyls) are some of the most common "invaders" to sneak into the body. These chemicals, widely used—and dumped into the environment—since the 1930s, find their way into our air, our water and our food.

PCBs, even in extremely low doses, can cause ill health, and they are a known cause of cancer in animals.

Over 90 percent of all Americans have detectable levels of PCBs stored in their fatty tissues.

Researchers from Japan have found that vitamin A may be a "guardian" in this instance, too. In one study on vitamin A and PCBs, researchers fed two groups of rats PCBs for six weeks, but gave one group 3,400 I.U. of vitamin A. The vitamin A group "showed better growth" than the animals not on the vitamin.

The researchers then fed another group of rats PCBs and measured the vitamin A content of the rats' livers. They found a decrease in vitamin A "even at low PCB levels."

Citing these and other studies, the researchers concluded that "a large part of the symptoms" of PCB poisoning "were based on a vitamin A deficiency" caused by PCBs.

Vitamin A is needed to counter other pollutants, too, especially those that stress our lungs. Every day, epithelial cells lining the respiratory tract are killed by bacteria, poisonous gases and other airborne enemies, and every day they grow back, literally as good as new. Without this power to regenerate, our lungs wouldn't last long in the chemical soup that passes for air in modern cities.

How well the lungs can hold their own in the face of unrelenting assault means the difference between health and very serious disease. Here again, vitamin A is a nutrient that strengthens the fortress.

Some of the most impressive evidence of this protective ability has come from a study that brought vitamin A into action against a particularly destructive enemy of lung health—a noxious gas called nitrogen dioxide (NO_2).

If you've ever noticed a brownish cast to the smog smothering a city, you've seen NO_2. It comes from automobile exhaust and industrial wastes. It is contained in cigarette smoke and produced when coal or

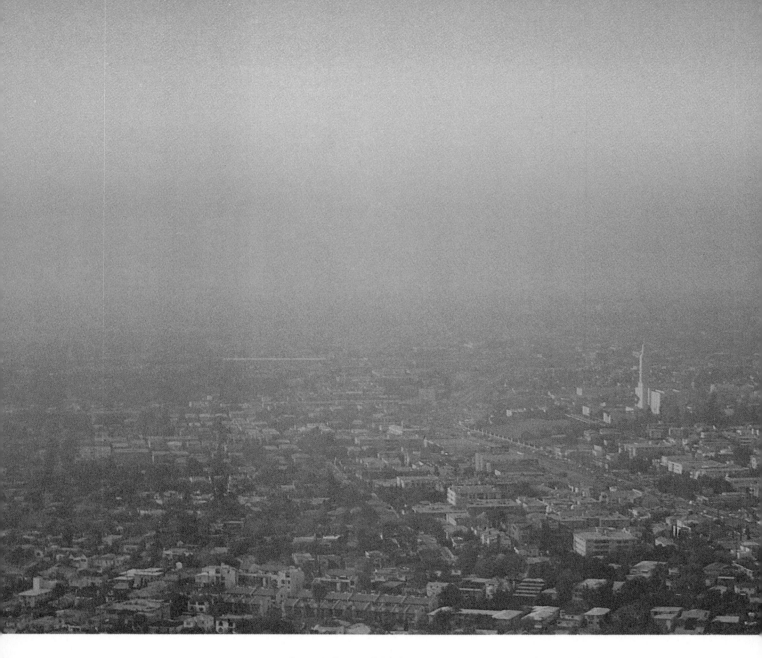

natural gas is burned for heat.

Laboratory tests have shown that NO_2 can damage lung tissue, producing the deteriorated state associated with emphysema. After exposure to NO_2, it has been found, animals are more susceptible to infections of the lung. (In human beings, air pollution in general has been linked to high rates of respiratory infections.)

What kind of protection can vitamin A offer against this poison gas? At the Delta Regional Primate Research Center of Tulane University, James C. S. Kim, D.V.M., Sc.D., exposed three groups of hamsters to NO_2 for five-hour periods once a week for eight weeks. The conditions, he explained, were "comparable not only to industrial pollution found in an urban-suburban environment, but also to the exposure of the respiratory tract of a habitual smoker."

The first group of hamsters received a diet lacking in vitamin A. The second got what Dr. Kim called a "vitamin A-adequate" diet. The third was fed a "vitamin A-high" diet—twice what the second group received. After the trial, the hamsters' lung tissues were examined.

Vitamin A-deficient animals, Dr. Kim noted, responded poorly to NO_2 exposure: "Rapid and often labored breathing appeared immediately and continued throughout the five hours. Recovery was slow." By the fifth week of the experiment, they had visibly started to decline. Microscopic examination of their lung tissues revealed severe damage.

Los Angeles is the smog capital of America, but many other cities have it almost as bad. To help your lungs combat this noxious mix of ozone, nitrogen dioxide and a host of other grimy ingredients, try vitamin A. It's a kind of internal gas mask.

The hamsters that received a vitamin A-adequate diet fared a good deal better. NO_2 made them breathe rapidly, but they showed no signs of distress and afterward their breathing quickly returned to normal. They remained in good condition throughout the eight weeks of the experiment—"healthy and alert." Their lungs showed no signs of pneumonia or the severe inflammation that had afflicted the deficient group. The gas had caused damage, certainly, but normal lung tissue had apparently grown back to repair it. The epithelial lining, for the most part, was intact and there were few abnormal cells.

The animals that received double doses of vitamin A survived their polluted environment equally well.

Observation and microscopic examination showed them to be much like the vitamin A-adequate group.

Too little vitamin A in the face of NO_2 exposure can raise the risk of disease, Dr. Kim believes. "Without vitamin A, ciliated epithelium doesn't form. Instead, you get squamous cells—precarcinoma-type cells. You get abnormal mucus cells, which mean clogging in the respiratory tract and danger of infection. If the epithelium doesn't form properly, it can lead to emphysema and chronic bronchitis."

His findings should be of special interest to commuters, Dr. Kim says, because they subject themselves to conditions much like those of his experiment. "If you commute, you have intermittent exposure to NO_2.

You may be exposed to urban pollution for five hours, eight hours, then you come back to your house in the suburbs, where the air is cleaner. The next day you go back to the city. The epithelium in the lung has to repair itself accordingly, after each exposure."

Vitamin A can help the lungs adapt to this less than perfect world, Dr. Kim says, "but a commuter who doesn't get enough vitamin A is going to suffer."

BUFFER AGAINST CANCER

The evidence has been piling up higher than a bumper crop of sweet potatoes: Eating foods high in vitamin A just may be your buffer against cancer.

It's long been recognized that vitamin A is essential in maintaining the structural integrity of cells. And scientists know that there is a significant relationship between the effects of vitamin A on the cells of the epithelium and the development of cancer in those tissues. These particular forms of cancer, which include cancer of the bronchial tubes and throat, the stomach, intestine, uterus, kidneys, bladder, testes, prostate and the skin, account for more than half of all cancers in both men and women.

Michael B. Sporn, M.D., of the National Cancer Institute, a leading authority on the connection between vitamin A and cancer, explains that an important factor in vitamin A's cancer-preventing potential may be its control of a specific action in the body called cell differentiation.

"Differentiation is the process that makes the cell what it is, that allows it to carry out the normal functions of a cell. When a cell dedifferentiates, those functions are lost, and the cell enters a primitive state. Its behavior becomes similar to that of a cancer cell. Proper maturation does not take place in cells that are dedifferentiated. Vitamin A is known to be involved in the maturation process, and that's why we chose vitamin A, rather than some other vitamin, to study.

"Many of the body's hormones are also involved in the proper maturation of cells, and vitamin A has the same hormonelike effects, but unlike a hormone, it cannot be manufactured in the body. The body must get its vitamin A from outside sources, and if it doesn't, the cells dedifferentiate, entering a state similar to that of cancerous cells."

Since vitamin A is the key to normal cellular controls, the logical step for researchers has been to feed laboratory animals vitamin A-enriched diets to test their resistance to cancer. The first important studies were carried out in 1967, with hamsters. Those fed vitamin A showed a marked ability to suppress the development of cancer. In other studies performed in the past decade vitamin A and its chemical derivatives have been shown to block the effects of cancer-causing substances in the lungs, stomach, bladder, breasts, skin and reproductive system of laboratory animals.

No one is saying that cancer is *caused* by not getting enough vitamin A or foods rich in that vitamin. But there is a lot of research indicating that those who eat green and yellow vegetables on a routine basis are a lot more successful at avoiding cancer or beating it down than those who don't.

As we've already mentioned, the protective factor is beta-carotene, a natural pigment found in certain vegetables and even some fruits. Once inside our bodies, carotene is converted to usable vitamin A.

One of the many important research projects concerning beta-carotene was carried out by Richard B. Shekelle, Ph.D., of Rush-Presbyterian-St. Luke's Medical Center in Chicago. Dr. Shekelle's study actually began as a long-term investigation into coronary heart disease in 2,107 workers at the Western Electric Company in Chicago. One aspect of the study was to record what the men ate every day. When it came to plotting vitamin A intake, Dr. Shekelle and his colleagues decided to divide the vitamin intake into that which came from animal sources (whole milk, liver, cream, butter and cheese) and that which came from fruits and vegetables rich in beta-carotene.

Over the next 19 years, 33 of the men developed lung cancer—all

Can Vitamin A Block Out the Majority of Cancers?

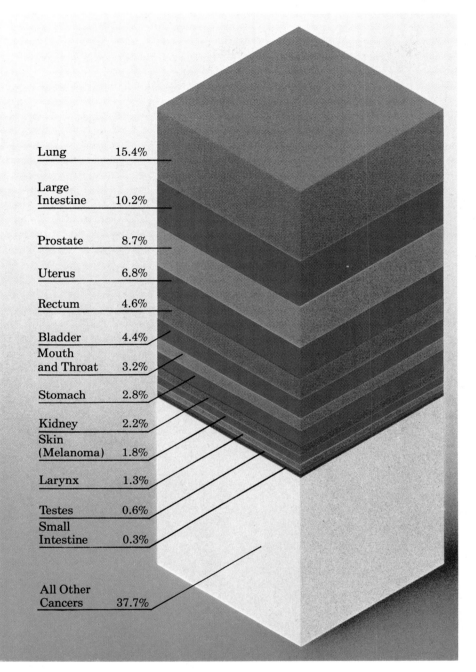

Lung	15.4%
Large Intestine	10.2%
Prostate	8.7%
Uterus	6.8%
Rectum	4.6%
Bladder	4.4%
Mouth and Throat	3.2%
Stomach	2.8%
Kidney	2.2%
Skin (Melanoma)	1.8%
Larynx	1.3%
Testes	0.6%
Small Intestine	0.3%
All Other Cancers	37.7%

Over 60 percent of all cancers have one thing in common: they involve epithelial tissue, the protective layer of cells that lines all the body's tissues, inside and out (the skin, for instance, is epithelial tissue, as is the lining of the digestive tract). Vitamin A strengthens epithelial tissue, and experts believe that if we ate a diet rich in the nutrient, all these cancers might be prevented.

related to cigarette smoking. However, Dr. Shekelle and his colleagues noticed something else very significant in those who developed lung cancer. The rate was highest in those who ate the least amounts of beta-carotene foods and lowest in those who ate the greatest amounts. The result: an 8-to-1 difference in risk between the lowest and highest groups.

Clearly, prevention is the name of the game. "No human population at risk for development of cancer should be allowed to remain in a vitamin A-deficient state," Dr. Sporn has written. Considering the relatively low cost of supplementation of the diet with a minimum daily requirement of vitamin A, he adds, "this is certainly a goal which should be met for the entire population."

4

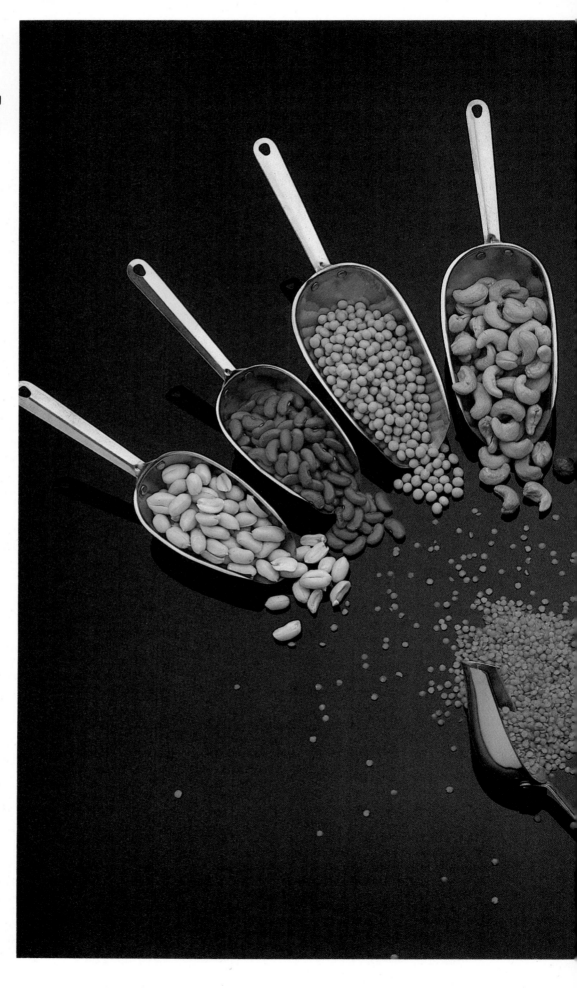

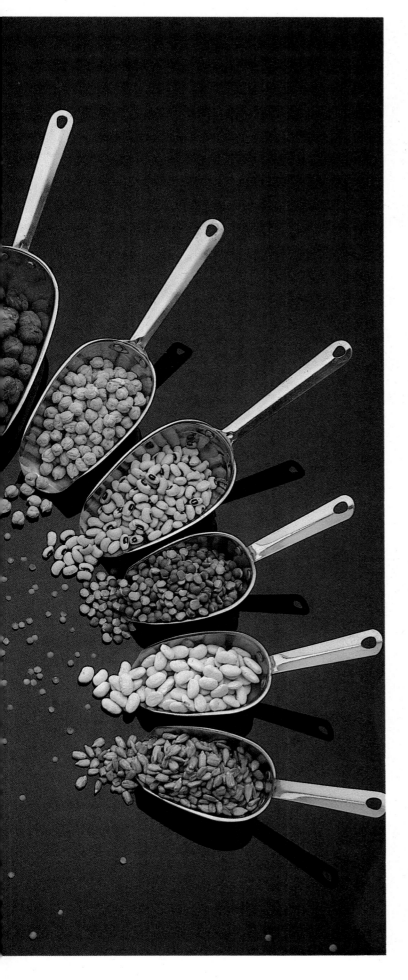

The B Complex Vitamins

Together the B vitamins make up the roster of a winning nutritional team for health.

Teamwork is something special. It's a cooperative magic that happens when talented individuals get together and bring out the best in each other. Whether it's a baseball team that wins the World Series or a singing group that tops the charts, the team simply wouldn't work as well—or might not work at all—if someone decided to take the day off.

Just like the B vitamins.

Thiamine, riboflavin, niacin, vitamins B_6 and B_{12} and folate—along with the lesser known but still vital nutrients pantothenate, para-aminobenzoic acid (PABA), inositol, biotin and choline—comprise what we call the B complex vitamins, which give us a lot more health mileage if each and every one is included in our diet.

A lack of all or some of them can lead to serious ailments, both mental and physical. But adding the B's to the diet can chase the blues, eradicate itchy dermatitis, prevent premenstrual tension, heal the heart and bring on the Sandman for insomniacs. Some of the B vitamins have even worked to cure difficult and devastating mental diseases, such as schizophrenia. And that's only a sampling of the therapeutic powers of the B family. Roger Williams, Ph.D., D.Sc., a University of Texas chemist and pioneer vitamin researcher, places special emphasis on the teamwork principle.

"Each B vitamin fits into different parts of the metabolic machinery of every living cell. And like cogs on a wheel, each has a specialized function," he explains.

But to prevent or cure disease, Dr. Williams explains, nutrients must also work cooperatively.

"When human beings are fortunate enough to maintain health by consuming wholesome food, this is accomplished by reason of the fact that they consume regularly *every one* of about 40 nutritional essentials .... We utilize in our bodies all nutritional elements simultaneously every day," a paper co-authored by Dr. Williams points out.

Unfortunately, try as we might, many of us can't meet all our B vitamin needs from food alone. Before modern food processing, it was reasonably possible to eat hearty and satisfy B vitamin needs. But when white bread became the staff of life, the nutrient team came up short on a number of key players.

"Milling removes a significant portion of wheat's B vitamins," Paul LaChance, Ph.D., professor of nutrition at Rutgers University, says. "What gets added back and what gets left behind depend both on federal regulation and company policy."

He explains that niacin and thiamine are restored to roughly the same amount as would be found in whole wheat. And enriched white flour actually has more riboflavin in it than does the original grain.

"Enrichment helped eradicate beriberi and pellagra," notes Dr. LaChance. "The public health benefits have been very real."

But he admits that white-as-the-driven-snow refined flour is but a pale echo of the whole wheat original. Depending on the degree of refinement, significant amounts of B_6, folate, pantothenate and other nutrients may be lost—and not restored.

Since enrichment is partial at best, it offers a false sense of security. Better by far would be a diet rich in complete B vitamin sources.

Liver, milk products, whole grains, lean meats and many vegetables are tasty ways to eat your way to vitamin self-sufficiency.

And think about adding a B complex supplement as a kind of nutritional insurance.

B Vitamin-Rich Recipe: Time-Saver Drink

Makes 2 cups

½ cup Time-Saver Drink Mix *(see recipe below)*
1 banana
1 teaspoon blackstrap molasses
2 teaspoons brewer's yeast

¼ teaspoon ground cinnamon
1 cup ice water

Combine all ingredients in blender and process.

Time-Saver Drink Mix
Makes 5½ cups

Prepare this nutrient-rich mix ahead of time and avoid the early-morning grinding and combining hassle.

½ cup sunflower seeds
½ cup sesame seeds
½ cup almonds
½ cup oat groats or oat flakes
½ cup carob powder
½ cup wheat germ
1 cup powdered skim milk
1½ cups soy powder (not flour)

Grind the seeds, nuts and oats very fine. Add remaining ingredients and mix thoroughly. Store in glass jars in refrigerator or freezer.

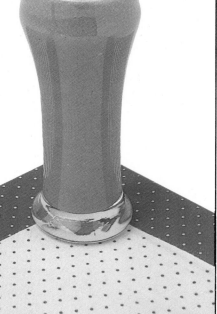

THIAMINE FOR STEADY NERVES

Without thiamine (vitamin B_1), the brain and nervous system collapse. Arms and legs lose their coordination. Eye muscles freeze in paralysis. The mind blackens into amnesia, coma and eventual death. Of course, that's the worst scenario, caused by an *extreme* deficiency. But even a *slight* deficiency of thiamine wounds the brain. Poor memory, irritability, depression, lack of initiative, insomnia, inability to concentrate—those are the symptoms of a mild thiamine deficiency, symptoms too often diagnosed as senility or neurosis.

In one study, reported in the *International Journal of Vitamin and Nutrition Research*, researchers compared the thiamine levels of 18 women with senility with those of 10 healthy people. Fifteen of the 18

The Best Food Sources of B Complex Vitamins

Food	Portion	Thiamine (mg.)	Riboflavin (mg.)	Niacin (mg.)	B₆ (mg.)	B₁₂ (mcg.)	Folate (mcg.)
Beef, lean	3 oz.	0.1	0.2	3.9	0.2	1.4	3
Brewer's yeast	1 tbsp.	1.3	0.3	3.0	0.2	0	313
Chicken, white meat	3 oz.	0.1	0.1	10.6	0.5	0.3	3
Chick-peas, dried	¼ cup	0.2	0.1	1.0	0.3	0	100
Egg, hard-cooked	1	0	0.1	0	0.1	0.7	24
Flour, rye	¼ cup	0.2	0.1	0.9	0.1	0	17
Flour, whole wheat	¼ cup	0.2	0	1.3	0.1	0	16
Kidney beans, dried	¼ cup	0.2	0.1	1.1	0.2	0	62
Kidney, beef	3 oz.	0.4	4.1	9.1	0.2	19.0	54
Liver, beef	3 oz.	0.2	3.6	14.0	0.5	49.0	123
Liver, chicken	3 oz.	0.1	1.5	3.8	0.5	16.5	654
Milk, whole	1 cup	0.1	0.4	0.2	0.1	0.9	12
Navy beans, dried	¼ cup	0.3	0.1	1.2	0.3	0	66
Peanuts, chopped	¼ cup	0.1	0.1	6.2	0.1	0	38
Rice, brown, raw	¼ cup	0.2	0	2.4	0.3	0	8
Salmon steak	3 oz.	0.2	0.1	8.4	0.6	3.0	18
Soybeans, dried	¼ cup	0.6	0.2	1.2	0.4	0	90
Sunflower seeds, dried	¼ cup	0.7	0.1	2.0	0.5	0	85
Swiss cheese	2 oz.	0	0.2	0.1	0.1	1.0	4
Wheat germ, toasted	1 tbsp.	0.1	0.1	0.3	0.1	0	25

NOTE: Meat, fish and poultry items are cooked.

women had "suboptimal blood levels" of thiamine, while all 10 of the healthy people had normal levels.

In another study, the average thiamine level of 65 neurotic patients was compared with that of 49 healthy people. The neurotic group had a level 58 percent lower than the healthy group. And in a study of the thiamine levels of 154 British psychiatric patients, researchers found more thiamine deficiencies among those patients with severe disorders (such as schizophrenia) than among those with milder illnesses.

Some researchers believe that a thiamine deficiency causes mental problems by cutting down the availability of serotonin, a chemical in the brain that helps regulate emotions. Yet no matter what the mechanism, it's good to know that thiamine supplementation can soothe jangled nerves that are crying out for the nutrient.

One study, reported by British physicians, concerned a group of psychiatric patients, among them "two elderly women . . . with severe clouding of consciousness suggestive of Wernicke's encephalopathy [a degenerative brain disease associated with alcoholism]." The two women had other psychiatric symptoms as well, but "in both cases, following [intravenous thiamine], the clouding cleared in 48 hours."

In another, even more remarkable case, 20 patients with such symptoms as sleep disturbances, personality changes (sometimes hostility), fevers of unknown origin, intermittent diarrhea and lack of appetite were studied. As the researchers pointed out in the *American Journal of Clinical Nutrition,* many of these symptoms "would represent a trap for the unwary physician since he would be unable to find any objective physical sign

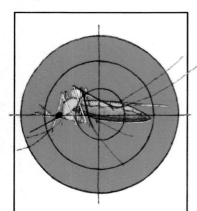

B₁ Bombs Mosquitoes

Some people swear that an extra dose of thiamine repels pesky mosquitoes. Many scientists don't buy that assertion. To find out the facts, researchers at Lake Superior State College in Michigan had 60 volunteers take either a B₁ supplement or a fake pill. Then the volunteers went outdoors and logged "bites received" for a few days. The result: Some found B₁ actually *did* repel the bugs— which means that thiamine might be worth a try.

other than variations of normal, which would be easily classed as the effects of a chronic state of anxiety. Thus some of the physical signs that we observed were the classical signs which have generally become associated with 'neurotic tension.'" Of course, these symptoms were not life-threatening, but they were "nevertheless debilitating and extremely frustrating since many of [the patients] had already received conventional therapy unsuccessfully."

Could low thiamine be the culprit here? Apparently so, for the researchers reported that "all of the 20 patients noticed marked symptomatic improvement or lost their symptoms completely after thiamine supplementation." It's also interesting that many of the patients had been consuming large quantities of junk foods, notably soft drinks.

A DEFICIENCY AMONG TEENAGERS

Derrick Lonsdale, M.D., of Cleveland, is a pediatrician who sees thiamine deficiency regularly in patients who are addicted to cola and empty-calorie foods. He studied a group of 20 people, most of whom were teenagers. Typically, they disdained breakfast and followed the general teenage pattern of eating: wolfing down lunch, looting the pantry for cake and cookies and washing these naked calories down with more naked calories in the form of soda pop. By suppertime, still sated from their after-school binge, they weren't interested in solid food.

Dr. Lonsdale's subjects exhibited two definite kinds of symptoms. All of them suffered from "neurotic" symptoms such as depression, insomnia, chest pain, recurrent fever and chronic fatigue. Several of the teenagers, in addition, were prone to bewildering "Dr. Jekyll and Mr. Hyde" personality changes, becoming suddenly sensitive to criticism, aggressive and hostile.

Blood tests indicated that every member of this group suffered from a relative thiamine deficiency.

Twelve of the 20 reported diets high in junk food. That made sense.

Thiamine is a catalyst in the burning of carbohydrates. When there's too much carbohydrate and not enough thiamine, Dr. Lonsdale theorized, the excess unburned carbohydrate tends to overstimulate the brain. The body experiences this imbalance as a thiamine deficiency, and shows some of the nervous symptoms of early beriberi.

"It has long been known," Dr. Lonsdale notes, "that a high-carbohydrate diet is most dangerous in the presence of a thiamine deficiency." He adds, "There is evidence for widespread nutritional deficiency in the U.S."

Thiamine supplementation (between 150 and 600 milligrams per day, a level that should be used only under a doctor's supervision) relieved the symptoms of every member of Dr. Lonsdale's study group. He concluded that a lot of the personality disruption and apparent mental problems of American adolescents could simply be the result of thiamine deficiency. "None of them [the teenagers] or their parents had the slightest notion that their symptoms might be related to their diets," Dr. Lonsdale says.

THIAMINE HELPS THE HEART

Complaining of severe shortness of breath that had steadily worsened over the preceding 30 hours, a 40-year-old Kansas City, Kansas, man was admitted to the Veterans' Administration Medical Center there. His hands and feet and the area around his mouth had turned blue, his heart was racing and his blood pressure had fallen dramatically. The doctors who treated him, learning that he was a heavy beer drinker, made a shrewd diagnosis and injected thiamine.

His blood pressure began rising almost immediately and he eventually recovered completely.

The man was a victim of what the doctors, writing in the medical journal *Chest,* called "acute pernicious beriberi heart disease." They explained that it's caused by chronic thiamine deficiency due to drinking. Over the long haul, thiamine shortages can cause a weakening of the heart muscle and, eventually, cardiac failure.

Few Americans die of beriberi heart disease. But *many* Americans have heart problems—problems they might solve if they upped their intake of thiamine.

When researchers measured the thiamine blood levels of over 125 elderly people, they found that 32 percent were deficient in thiamine—and that heart pain was more common among those with a deficiency.

In a study at the University of Alabama Medical Center in Birmingham, researchers measured the daily thiamine intake of 74 people, and then had them fill out a questionnaire in which they listed their cardiovascular (heart and circulatory system) complaints.

Dividing the people into high-intake and low-intake groups, they found that those with a low intake of thiamine had almost twice as many cardiovascular complaints.

A study from Japan has provided more proof that thiamine strengthens the heart. There, in the ten days before their open heart surgery, one group of patients received thiamine, while another group of patients did not. When their hearts were artificially stopped to perform the operation, only 10 percent of the thiamine group had abnormal heart spasms, compared with 30 percent of the other group. And, when their hearts were revived at the end of the operation, 30 percent of the thiamine group had heart spasms, compared with 95 percent of the other group.

RIBOFLAVIN KEEPS YOU IN THE PINK

If your tongue is moderate in size, a nice pink color, smooth around the edges without indentations showing where your teeth touch it, or if it resembles the tongue of a healthy child, chances are you are well supplied with B vitamins, including riboflavin, also known as vitamin B_2.

But if your tongue has a purplish cast, more like fuchsia or magenta than pink roses, then indeed, you may need more riboflavin. And even before your tongue changed color, you may have experi-

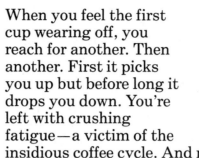

Coffee Scalds Your Thiamine

When you feel the first cup wearing off, you reach for another. Then another. First it picks you up but before long it drops you down. You're left with crushing fatigue—a victim of the insidious coffee cycle. And maybe a victim of thiamine deficiency.

Along with excessive sugar and alcohol, too much coffee seriously depletes the body's stores of thiamine. The result: jittery nerves, irritability and a feeling that you're out of control. Maybe you go around slamming cabinets. Or sink into depression at the prospect of doing everyday tasks.

Coffee's role as a thiamine thief was uncovered in a study presented in the *International Journal of Vitamin and Nutrition Research*. Twenty-five students at the University of Zurich in Switzerland agreed to drink a quart of coffee over a 3-hour period. Eight days later they drank an equal amount of water. Urine specimens taken after each session revealed that on the average there was nearly 50 percent less thiamine in the urine after coffee ingestion than after drinking water. Coffee apparently destroyed much of the thiamine obtained in the diet. And drinking decaffeinated coffee—or tea, for that matter—isn't a way out. They destroy thiamine, too.

enced nervousness and digestive disturbances, which are also associated with riboflavin deficiency, with unusual frequency.

Maybe you also have cracks at the corners of your mouth, lines radiating from your lips, oily hair, blurred vision, a tendency to whip out your sunglasses at the first ray of golden sun, frequent tearing of the eyes, red, inflamed eyelids or flaky areas around your nose, eyebrows or

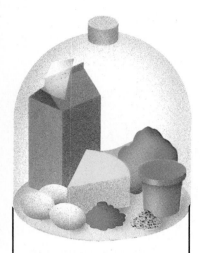

Retain That Riboflavin

Riboflavin is as sensitive as a prima donna. It's easily destroyed by exposure to light, as when milk is stored in glass jars. It is also easily destroyed by cooking, because it's water soluble. Here are some tips to preserve it:

Don't leave bottled milk out too long. Steam your vegetables; cooking them in large amounts of water for long periods of time butchers riboflavin. During cleaning, avoid soaking vegetables and fruits in large quantities of water.

hairline. Many of these conditions respond to riboflavin and are due to a dietary deficiency of this nutrient.

You may be consuming what you think is a well-balanced diet, and still suffer a deficiency of riboflavin. This water-soluble nutrient is quickly destroyed by light and by drugs like antibiotics, oral contraceptives and tranquilizers; it is also lost in sweat, urine and tears. As an enzyme activator, riboflavin is so busy that it is sometimes completely used up before it has completed its metabolic chores. And that's too bad, because riboflavin not only combines with proteins to form a number of essential enzymes necessary for the transport of oxygen, it also participates in the respiration of every single cell.

And if that's not enough to convince you of how very essential riboflavin is, consider this true account:

Just before her second birthday, a very ill little girl named Christina was brought to the Medical College of Georgia in Augusta. For no apparent reason, the child seemed to be losing her abilities to see, hear and walk, and she had life-threatening anemia. She was put in the care of three doctors: Patricia Hartlage, M.D., Dorothy Hahn, M.D., and Robert Leshner, M.D.

The doctors were puzzled. In spite of an adequate diet and even a daily multivitamin with iron, Christina's anemia wouldn't quit. "We were keeping her alive with transfusions," Dr. Hartlage says. "She was a pretty sick little girl."

Searching for an effective treatment for the anemia, the doctors turned to B vitamins. Under the microscope, Christina's red blood cells were disfigured by "funny little bubbles" called vacuoles; B vitamins are known to promote the production of healthy red blood cells.

The doctors narrowed the choices down to vitamin B_6, thiamine and riboflavin, and decided to give Christina high doses of each of them individually, for one month each. They tried B_6 and thiamine, but neither had any effect. Then, almost as a last resort, they gave her riboflavin. Five days later, "Whammo!" recalls Dr. Hartlage. "Christina started to produce healthy red blood cells."

"We just happened to try riboflavin last," Dr. Hahn explains. "We gave her the vitamins in sequence. Riboflavin was the last we tried, and lo and behold, she responded to it. If we had tried riboflavin first, we would never have known whether thiamine or pyridoxine [B_6] would have worked or not."

Even more amazingly, riboflavin began to reverse the neurological damage done to Christina's eyesight and hearing. Riboflavin deficiency is known to affect the blood and skin, but not the nervous system in humans. "We haven't been able to find any similar reports in the medical literature," Dr. Hahn says. "We've talked to hematologists, neurologists and pediatricians."

Christina's illness was an extreme and unique case. Her diet contained all the riboflavin most of us would need, but she had a rare need for large amounts of it. Her response to riboflavin and riboflavin alone, however, shows that the vitamin has what Dr. Leshner calls a "niche of its own" among the B vitamins.

Riboflavin's remarkable effect on little Christina's blood was due to the fact that the nutrient lengthens the lives of red blood cells and boosts the role of folate in the production of new red blood cells in bone marrow. Riboflavin also seems to help maintain a high level of iron in red blood cells.

RED BLOOD CELLS AND RIBOFLAVIN

British researchers found that red blood cells in riboflavin-deficient people have a shorter life span than normal. The deficiency in each cell seems to weaken its ability to resist damage from highly reactive oxidants. The cells die before their time and are filtered out of the blood.

A researcher from the University of Ghana in West Africa—where diets are commonly low in riboflavin—found a special relationship between riboflavin and folate. Knowing that folate is responsible for the production of red blood cells, he found that folate works much better if it's reinforced by a dose of riboflavin.

"Riboflavin may be exerting its effect through its involvement in folate metabolism," he noted in the *International Journal of Vitamin and Nutrition Research*.

The researcher also found that, by a separate process, "riboflavin is involved in the absorption and utilization of dietary iron" in the blood. He suggests that riboflavin supplements should accompany iron therapy, adding that "in pregnancy, iron and folate deficiencies are common and the addition of riboflavin to iron and folate used in treatment may be advisable."

With that in mind, every expectant mother should include a good riboflavin source such as yogurt or brewer's yeast in her daily routine. Riboflavin has been shown to relieve the muscular cramps of pregnancy, and it seems to have a detoxifying effect on pollutants and drugs that can seriously affect the baby.

Currently, some scientists are suggesting that people afflicted with cataracts should realize that they, too, may have an increased need for riboflavin. At the University of Alabama, Harold W. Skalka, M.D., and Josef Prchal, M.D., are two researchers pursuing a scientific lead that might make some of the 400,000 cataract operations performed every year in the United States unnecessary.

"Riboflavin might not prevent cataracts," Dr. Skalka explains, "but it may be able to help retard their formation. That is, instead of a person developing cataracts at 50, you could hold it back to age 60 or 70 or 80 in some cases." (See "Riboflavin: The Eyes Should Have It.")

It's clear that growing children, pregnant women and cataract victims are not the only ones who need riboflavin. We all need riboflavin.

Jack M. Cooperman, Ph.D., director of nutritional education at New York Medical College in Valhalla, has studied riboflavin levels in several groups of Americans. He says, "In this country, 60 percent of our riboflavin intake comes from milk or skim milk and other dairy products such as yogurt and cheese." He has found that people who don't consume much milk—such as urban teenagers—tend to be deficient in riboflavin.

Riboflavin: The Eyes Should Have It

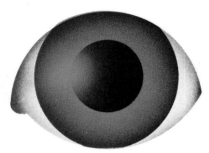

Patients over 50 with Cataracts

34% Deficient in Riboflavin

Patients over 50 without Cataracts

0% Deficient in Riboflavin

When a team of researchers from the University of Alabama measured the level of riboflavin in the blood of people over 50 with and without cataracts, they made a "striking finding": "the total absence of riboflavin deficiency in our older . . . patients with clear lenses." That means getting enough riboflavin might protect against cataracts. How can you make sure to get a preventive amount? Riboflavin supplements could be your best bet, say the researchers.

In a study of 210 white, Hispanic-American and black youths between the ages of 13 and 19 in New York City, Dr. Cooperman found that 26 percent were deficient in riboflavin. The teenagers with the highest levels were those who drank the most milk—up to 3 cups a day—and those with the lowest vitamin levels drank the least—1 cup a week. He found that black youths were especially susceptible to riboflavin deficiency. As a group, they often get cramps or diarrhea from milk and tend to avoid it, he reported in the *American Journal of Clinical Nutrition*.

Few people are seriously short of riboflavin, Dr. Cooperman says, but many may be marginally deficient and may suffer subtly. "With a marginal deficiency, no one knows exactly what the symptoms might be. Children may fail to grow properly. Adults may feel slightly ill. They might not be able to do a full day's work. They'll be mildly anemic and lackadaisical. That's all we know right now."

NIACIN MAKES LIFE NICER

Pellagra, the niacin deficiency disease, is almost unheard of in Western countries today. A quartet of symptoms, known as the four D's, tended to follow one another in this order: dermatitis in areas exposed to the sun, diarrhea, dementia and then death.

The Niacin Flush

If you find yourself blushing furiously and feeling all hot and itchy, it could be that supplement of nicotinic acid you just took. Niacin comes in 2 forms, nicotinic acid and niacinamide. When you take 100 milligrams or more of nicotinic acid, chemicals are released into your bloodstream, widening your blood vessels, and blood rushes to your skin. Hence, the so-called niacin flush. Fortunately, it's harmless and fades quickly. If you'd prefer to avoid the reaction, take no more than 50 milligrams of nicotinic acid at any one time.

That's because the sensitive, vital layers of tissue in the skin, tongue, intestines and nervous system depend very heavily on certain biochemical reactions that, in turn, depend very heavily on the availability of niacin.

A milder deficiency of niacin could cause, according to some medical researchers, such "everyday" problems as dermatitis, irritability and arthritis. Today niacin deficiencies don't usually progress much beyond the early stages, but they can be very unpleasant just the same.

William Kaufman, M.D., Ph.D., of Stratford, Connecticut, was a pioneer in the use of niacin therapy for subclinical pellagra. He explains, "When I began practicing medicine in 1941, before the compulsory enrichment of cereal products, I realized that there was something going on that was a bit unusual. I found it striking that patient after patient came in with a group of symptoms which were quite similar. They might have other symptoms besides. But in these certain symptoms, such as the lack of ability to concentrate, depression, irritability, joint complaints, excessive fatigue, bloating and intestinal complaints, there was fingerprint similarity.

"I began tabulating symptoms that these men, women and children had and very soon recognized that this strange syndrome was probably a form of pellagra, or niacin deficiency, that had not yet reached the degree of severity to cause the classic combination of skin rash, diarrhea and dementia.

"I reasoned if this was a form of pellagra, then niacinamide—which had then just been discovered as a preventative—might provide useful treatment. [Niacin comes in two forms, niacinamide and nicotinic acid.]

"I prescribed it, and patients would return a few days later and . . . I didn't believe it! They looked different. They acted different. They told me that their symptoms had vanished, they felt a new zest for life. I decided to test it. I gave a few of these improved patients calcium tablets instead of niacinamide. They were unaware of the change. At the end of ten days they were right back

to where they had been when they first saw me. When they resumed niacinamide treatment, they once again improved."

HELP FOR ARTHRITIS SYMPTOMS

Over the years, Dr. Kaufman has found that this member of the B complex produces remarkable results in relieving the pain and stiffness of arthritis. Dr. Kaufman has found that some of his patients need, in addition to niacinamide, "the whole B complex, especially thiamine, B_6 and B_{12}" and vitamin C, taken in divided doses throughout the day.

Niacinamide, says Dr. Kaufman, does not cure arthritis but rather controls the pain. The dosage must be supervised by a physician, he says, adding that "the daily dose I have prescribed since 1944 usually ranges from 900 to 4,000 milligrams a day in divided doses." An added benefit for his patients was an improved sense of balance.

NIACIN AND SCHIZOPHRENIA

You begin to hallucinate, seeing what isn't there and hearing voices when no one speaks. If it's not too severe, you know you're hallucinating. But if it's worse, you can't tell what's real and what's not. Your thoughts are bizarre and illogical, perhaps paranoid, and you act on them. You might think there's a plot against you. You might think you're God. You might talk of suicide and, very possibly, commit it.

Such are the characteristics of schizophrenia, a disease whose victims take up 25 percent of all hospital beds in America. But there's lots of proof that schizophrenics can be healed with nutrition—and niacin figures prominently in the picture. Thousands of schizophrenics have already been cured with niacin therapy.

A lack of niacin can actually cause madness. Soon after processors of white flour began fortifying it with niacin, 10 percent of all state hospital patients in the South were "cured." They had been diagnosed as schizophrenics, but they actually had pellagra. Some of the mental symptoms of pellagra—hallucinations and paranoia—perfectly mimic schizophrenia.

"If all the niacin were removed from our food, everyone would be psychotic in one year," says Abram Hoffer, M.D., a psychiatrist in British Columbia.

In 1952, Dr. Hoffer and a colleague gave niacin to eight schizophrenic patients. They immediately improved. Continuing the study, the doctors checked their patients' progress for the next 15 years. All were well 15 years later—and all were still taking niacin.

Schizophrenia can last a lifetime or a few weeks. Many patients walk out of state hospitals only to return. To see if niacin could keep schizophrenics permanently out of hospitals, Dr. Hoffer gave 73 hospitalized schizophrenics niacin and compared them with 98 who were not taking niacin. During the next three years, only 7 of the niacin patients had to be readmitted to a hospital, while 47 of the other patients were readmitted.

Doctors have also found niacin extremely effective for the treatment of depression and insomnia, especially when it is taken along with supplements of tryptophan.

In one study doctors gave tryptophan and niacin to 11 depressed patients. The doctors knew that, in some studies, depressed people took tryptophan but didn't get any better. They theorized that the tryptophan hadn't been metabolized properly, and that niacin would correct this problem. They were right. After only one month on tryptophan and niacin, the patients' blood levels of tryptophan rose almost 300 percent and their depression fell 38 percent.

According to H. L. Newbold, M.D., author of *Mega-Nutrients for Your Nerves* (Peter H. Wyden, 1975), "while most people feel better within days of beginning a niacin regimen, some require months to feel the benefits. It is especially important to give this vitamin a lengthy therapeutic trial because its potential benefits are so great."

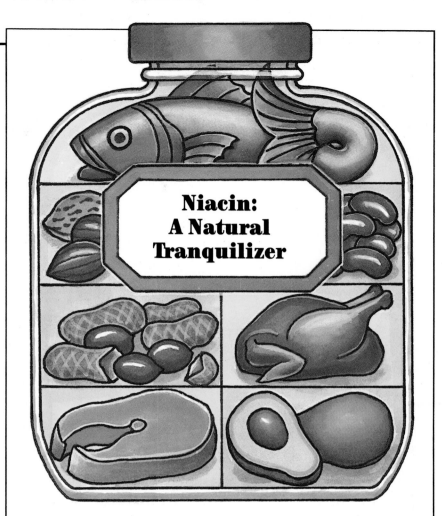

Niacin: A Natural Tranquilizer

Niacin is so soothing to the nervous system that even a research group from Hoffmann-La Roche Inc.—the well-known Swiss pharmaceutical company that manufactures Valium—has admitted that its effectiveness compares to that of certain tranquilizers. They've found that, like tranquilizers, niacinamide can induce "anticonflict" and "antiaggressive" feelings and that it relaxes muscles and helps relieve insomnia.

VITAMIN B₆ FOR COMMON AND UNCOMMON AILMENTS

Every vitamin has its limitations. Vitamin B_6 will not walk the dog, chauffeur the kids or do windows. But scientists are finding that B_6—pyridoxine—may do a lot of other things that might previously have been considered impossible. Research indicates that vitamin B_6 is tackling not only some common medical ailments, but some extraordinarily uncommon maladies, as well.

For starters, B_6 is essential for A-1 circulation. In the development of heart disease, one of the most important factors is the tendency of blood cells called platelets to clump together and form clots. (Doctors commonly treat heart patients with drugs that prevent clotting.) Abnormal clotting can cause serious problems not only in the heart, but also in the arteries feeding the brain and in the veins of the legs, kidneys and liver.

Elizabeth Kornecki, Ph.D., formerly of the thrombosis center at Temple University in Philadelphia, and Harold Feinberg, Ph.D., of the University of Illinois Medical Center in Chicago, have found that pyridoxal phosphate, one of the active forms of vitamin B_6 in the body, inhibits the action of a number of the chemicals that cause platelets to stick together in the bloodstream.

Adenosine diphosphate (ADP) is one of the platelet-aggregating chemicals that B_6 acts to inhibit. ADP is contained in grainlike particles within the platelets. "A cloud of ADP is released into the blood," Dr. Feinberg explains. "The ADP makes the platelets in the blood adhesive to one another, and they form a plug which blocks the flow of blood out of the damaged vessel. That's a very simplified version of what happens, but it's accurate."

Other chemicals in the body that play a role in platelet aggregation include thrombin, collagen, epinephrine and arachidonic acid. It's a complex process and, obviously, it does not result in blood clots every time some slight injury occurs in a blood vessel. Problems arise only when abnormally sensitive platelets form clots that are not needed to stop bleeding. The tantalizing possibility, Dr. Feinberg says, is that "by simply altering our diets, we might end up with less reactive platelets, platelets which still form clots when necessary, but don't produce all this other trouble."

Dr. Kornecki and Dr. Feinberg have demonstrated that pyridoxal phosphate inhibits the action of ADP and partially interferes with platelet aggregation triggered by epinephrine and arachidonic acid. In another study, the researchers showed that B_6 also inhibits thrombin directly.

Evidence of the vitamin's effectiveness is not confined to test-tube studies. Several years ago, researchers at Northwestern University and Temple University medical schools were able to directly test the effects of B_6 on platelet aggregation. Volunteers in the study were given just one dose of 100 milligrams of B_6. As expected, platelet aggregation was significantly reduced, in some cases not returning to normal levels for over two days after the B_6 was taken.

B_6 may also protect the circulatory system by preventing the buildup of cholesterol in the blood. One study with rats found that large doses of B_6 included in a high-fat, high-cholesterol diet reduced the accumulation of cholesterol in the blood usually produced by such a diet.

If you're older, you should take particular care to get enough vitamin B_6. Not only are the elderly more susceptible to heart problems, but also they often suffer from vitamin B_6 deficiencies. Of the older people tested in nursing homes, over 30 percent had abnormally low blood

Stop Gallstones with B_6

According to doctors at the Wilhelmina Hospital in Vienna, Austria, preventing gallstones may be as easy as a trip to your nearest grocery and health food stores. In a carefully controlled study, the bile from 22 gallbladder patients was evaluated 3 days after surgery. Later, the same patients were given 1 tablespoon of corn oil and 50 milligrams of vitamin B_6 at 7 P.M. and midnight on one day and at 4 A.M. the next day. Bile samples were again taken and tested to determine if there was any change in the cholesterol-dissolving capacity of the bile. (Gallstones are formed when cholesterol builds up in the bile.)

Remarkably, *all* the patients were better able to keep their cholesterol in solution and the bile of some patients was able to dissolve more cholesterol than before the administration of the corn oil and B_6.

levels of vitamin B_6, says the *Journal of the American Geriatrics Society*.

Women on the Pill also have an increased risk of developing heart problems, especially blood clots and atherosclerosis. Vitamin B_6 has already been used to correct depression and mood changes in women taking the Pill, symptoms that might be caused by a B_6 deficiency.

B_6, GOD'S GIFT TO WOMEN

Actually, a woman doesn't even have to be taking oral contraceptives to benefit from B_6. There is now lots of evidence that the symptoms of premenstrual syndrome (PMS) and menstrual tension—including acne, depression, breast pain and bloating—can be greatly relieved by taking extra vitamin B_6 for about a week to ten days before each menstrual period.

In an experiment conducted by gynecologists Joel T. Hargrove, M.D., of Columbia, Tennessee, and Guy E. Abraham, M.D., of Rolling Hills, California, 25 women suffering from moderate to severe premenstrual tension received either 500 milligrams of vitamin B_6 or a placebo (a fake, look-alike pill) for three consecutive menstrual cycles. Twenty-one of the 25 patients noticed a decrease in their symptoms while taking B_6, but not while taking the placebo.

Dr. Hargrove was not surprised by the results of his study. He has been prescribing B_6 to his patients for years, with great success. (The level of B_6 prescribed by Dr. Hargrove should be taken only under a physician's supervision.)

Doctors now believe that high estrogen levels after ovulation play some part in either an increased need for vitamin B_6 or a lower ability to absorb it, and the resulting deficiency leads to annoying premenstrual symptoms.

Women on the Pill for three years or longer may require even more B_6—especially if a future pregnancy is planned.

"After that much time on the Pill, B_6 reserves may be greatly reduced," says Avanelle Kirskey, Ph.D., professor of food and nutri-

tion at Purdue University. "If the intake of B_6 is not adequate to meet the needs of pregnancy and to overcome the possible depletion by previous use of oral contraceptives, both the mother and the fetus could suffer."

Pregnancy may trigger diabetes in susceptible women. And this reaction, too, has been traced in some cases to low levels of vitamin B_6. Glucose tolerance was improved greatly by taking 100 milligrams of the vitamin daily for two weeks, according to a report in the *American Journal of Obstetrics and Gynecology*. (Once again, this is a level of intake that requires a doctor's okay.)

Losses of B_6 in Processing

Food	Percent of Loss
Shredded wheat	38
Cracked wheat bread	49
Puffed wheat	57
Saltine crackers	62
Spaghetti	64
French bread	70
White bread	78
All-purpose flour	82
Cake flour	87

As the original wheat kernel is subjected to ever greater processing, more B_6 is destroyed until losses approach 90 percent.

Nutrition-oriented physicians have also used vitamin B₆ in the treatment (and prevention) of yet another condition of pregnancy — toxemia.

EXTRA ENERGY

But it's not just women who suffer when B levels go down. A deficiency can make anyone irritable, restless, depressed — or tired. One doctor who believes that B₆ increases our stamina is John H. Richardson, M.D., of Old Dominion University in Norfolk, Virginia. In a study with rats, he was able to show that animals supplemented with B₆ suffered less fatigue and had more endurance during exercise than animals on an unsupplemented diet.

Meanwhile, at the University of Oregon, scientists have also investi-gated the link between B₆ and exercise. "There is always an increase in the need for B₆ during physical stress," Frantisek Bartos, Ph.D., says. "People in general have a greater-than-RDA need for the vitamin, but in athletes the need is even more pronounced. We know that the amount of B₆ in a normal diet is not sufficient."

Dr. Bartos says that B₆ supplements have increased his own energy.

Mental energy may also be boosted by vitamin B₆, according to several reports. In one study, researchers at Northwick Park Hospital in England examined a number of patients admitted to the hospital's psychiatric unit. They observed that a lack of vitamin B₆ in some of the patients seemed linked with depression.

The researchers concluded "more attention should be paid to assessing the . . . pyridoxine status of the mentally ill in the hope of detecting and correcting deficiencies."

B₆: An Answer to Infertility

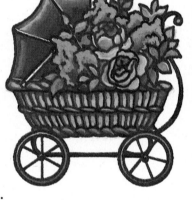

Women with unexplained infertility may find new hope for pregnancy in high doses of vitamin B₆, according to the findings of 2 gynecologists, Joel T. Hargrove, M.D., and Guy E. Abraham, M.D. Twelve of their 14 patients who had been infertile from 18 months to 7 years were finally able to conceive after vitamin B₆ therapy. The study participants, ranging in age from 23 to 31, had one thing in common: premenstrual tension. Vitamin B₆ was given daily in doses ranging from 100 to 800 milligrams, depending on the dose needed to relieve each patient's tension symptoms. (Use that level of intake only under a doctor's supervision.) Of the 13 pregnancies that resulted (one woman conceived twice), 11 occurred within the first 6 months of therapy, one occurred in the 7th month and the last occurred in the 11th month of the program.

HELPING AUTISTIC CHILDREN

A combination that can't be beat is B₆ and magnesium — especially for children with autism, a condition characterized by withdrawal, lack of interest in people and aversion to affection. These children are virtually alone in their own inner world.

But Bernard Rimland, Ph.D., director of the Institute for Child Behavior Research in San Diego, has seen amazing changes occur in these youngsters when they were given large amounts of B₆ — usually several hundred milligrams — along with magnesium.

In a study published in the *American Journal of Psychiatry*, Dr. Rimland and two medical colleagues described what happened when 16 autistic children stopped taking their supplements. The experiment was set up in such a way that neither the youngsters, their parents nor the doctors knew when the subjects were taking B₆ and magnesium and when they were taking worthless substitutes.

In 11 of the cases, the children's behavior gave the secret away. Their behavior deteriorated noticeably when they stopped taking the combination and rebounded just as sharply when they resumed. Without the supplements, the children refused to talk. They would whine and shake nervously, hide under blankets or retreat into their rooms. Interest and involvement in their surroundings shrank to a minimum.

But with B_6 and magnesium, those same youngsters began to talk more, read, ask questions and play games. They became calmer and better able to socialize with their friends and family.

In another study conducted in France, 52 children diagnosed as autistic were treated with B_6, magnesium, a combination of B_6 and magnesium, or a placebo. After four weeks the children were reexamined and their symptoms reevaluated. The combination of magnesium and B_6 was confirmed as effective for autistic symptoms, say the researchers. By contrast, when given separately these nutrients had no significant therapeutic effect.

Other studies have confirmed the effectiveness of B_6 in treating not only autism, but also other childhood problems such as hyperactivity and epileptic-type convulsions.

Incredibly, the list goes on: Vitamin B_6 also helps people who suffer from recurrent kidney stone formation, especially stones that are composed mainly of oxalates. And, since both magnesium and B_6 have been reported successful in preventing kidney stones in susceptible patients, scientists feel that B_6 increases the utilization of magnesium by aiding the transport of this mineral across cell membranes.

Diabetics, too, can reap the benefits of B_6. Studies at the Thordek Medical Center in Chicago have shown that a type of eye problem associated with diabetes may disappear with B_6 supplementation.

In addition, the eye disease gyrate atrophy may respond well to B_6 therapy, says Richard Weleber, M.D., of the University of Oregon Health Sciences Center in Portland. He and his colleagues report that some patients with the rare disease have a B_6 *dependency* (rather than a deficiency), which means they have an inherited need for large doses of the nutrient.

A LIGHT AT THE END OF THE CARPAL TUNNEL

One of the most exciting breakthroughs in recent years, though, is the use of vitamin B_6 to cure carpal tunnel syndrome, a neurological disorder causing pain and tingling in the hands and frequently in the arm and shoulder. The condition can progress to the point where a person becomes unable to carry even light objects.

For years, patients with this disorder were routinely subjected to hand surgery to relieve compression on the nerve. But it's no secret that the surgery may be only partially successful and that any relief gained is likely to be lost in a few months.

Now, permanent relief from carpal tunnel syndrome is perhaps only a B_6 supplement away, thanks to the research efforts of two Texans, John Ellis, M.D., and Karl Folkers, Ph.D., who have attained success using between 100 and 300 milligrams daily. Surgery, they say, should be a last-resort treatment for the condition. Like many scientists and nutritionists, Dr. Folkers believes the RDA of 2 milligrams is "far too low." He says, "I believe that an effective RDA would be around 25 milligrams, or possibly even 35 milligrams."

VITAMIN B_{12}: MORE THAN ANEMIA PROTECTION

Vitamin B_{12} is popularly known as a "pep vitamin," but its role is actually much more serious—and diverse— than that term implies. The plight of a young woman, described in the *South African Medical Association Journal*, is revealing.

The 35-year-old patient was in good health, was not taking any medications and had no physical problems except a very disturbing numbness in both legs, especially the left one, and a tendency to stumble to the left. She just couldn't walk straight. She'd developed an embarrassing, ducklike waddle, with her legs spread wide, because if she didn't waddle she'd lose her balance.

What worried her most was that

it seemed to be getting worse.

When she was examined by doctors at a hospital, they were perplexed. A battery of tests showed nothing abnormal.

So what was wrong with her? Was she crazy? She didn't think so, yet her condition continued to worsen after that first examination. She seemed to be losing control of her legs. She started having uncontrollable spasms in her thighs.

Then, two weeks after her first visit, her doctors tested a blood sample for levels of folate and

vitamin B_{12}. And at last they found something that *wasn't* normal: Her B_{12} levels were depleted severely.

The patient was given an injection of vitamin B_{12}—1,000 micrograms—and for the first time since her problem started she began to feel better. In a week she felt *much* better. Two months later, after receiving injections totaling 3,000 micrograms of vitamin B_{12}, all her symptoms had vanished.

This woman's story illustrates some of the essential chores vitamin B_{12} is forever performing inside our bodies, chores we rarely notice until they're left undone. B_{12} works tirelessly, keeping our nerves and blood in shape, maintaining healthy growth and even playing a role in the synthesis of DNA, the genetic blueprint we pass along to our children.

The abnormalities in the South African woman's blood and the neurological signs—the numbness, unsteadiness and muscle spasms—had made her doctors begin to suspect that a B_{12} deficiency might be the key.

They knew that because of the role of B_{12} in building the protein sheath that surrounds the nerve fibers and the spinal cord, a deficiency can result in a slow deterioration of the nerve tissue. And *that* begins to show up as numbness or prickly sensations in the extremities, burning feet, forgetfulness, depression and other mental problems.

B_{12} is also a supervisor in the red blood cell production department, which has to keep them rolling off the assembly line at about 200 million a minute. A B_{12} shortage there results in bloated, misshapen cells that are unable to carry oxygen (their main job in life), so you wind up pale, tired and anemic.

Vitamin B_{12} and its chemical cousins, known to scientists as cobalamins because they contain tiny amounts of the metal cobalt, are remarkable substances indeed. But if B_{12} is such a hot ticket, how come we don't hear all that much about it?

For one thing, the body needs only the tiniest amounts of vitamin B_{12} to function properly: The Recommended Dietary Allowance is 3 micrograms a day, or 3 *millionths* of a gram. For another, most people

Do Vegetarians Need Extra B₁₂?

Vitamin B_{12} occurs only in eggs, meat and dairy products, so some strict vegetarians take supplements of B_{12} as insurance. That's especially important for pregnant or nursing vegetarians, who should not leave B_{12} intake to chance because a deficiency passed on to the child may endanger the baby's life. But are supplements a must for *all* vegetarians? Well, a report in *New Scientist* says "there are still some vegans [vegetarians who eat no animal products whatsoever] who, while apparently eating nothing that can supply their B_{12} needs, have shown no serious deficiency over the years. We are being forced to conclude that these people are able to manufacture and absorb their own B_{12} in the gut [intestine]." Even so, if you're a vegan, look to possible sources of B_{12} such as fermented soy products like miso, soy sauce and tempeh.

have up to 1,000 times that amount squirreled away in their bodies. Strange as it sounds, vast colonies of busy, cobalamin-producing bacteria live right in your digestive tract, making B_{12} from every meal.

But even with all this extra B_{12} on hand, you may still wind up with a deficiency.

People who have had stomach or intestinal surgery are good candidates for vitamin B_{12} deficiency. Both hydrochloric acid and a substance called "intrinsic factor," which are secreted by the walls of the stomach, are necessary for B_{12} to be absorbed from food, but surgery interferes with these secretions and thus with the absorption of B_{12}. (Some people can get around this problem by taking large amounts of B_{12} in tablets or injections. Even without hydrochloric acid and intrinsic factor, about 1 percent of the B_{12} in a supplement would be absorbed through the small intestine.)

A number of drugs also can interfere with B_{12} absorption, including certain medications for high blood pressure, tuberculosis, Parkinson's disease, gout and excess cholesterol. Alcohol also adversely affects B_{12} absorption, just as it does the absorption of other B vitamins.

A deficiency of B_{12} may go undiagnosed for a long time, because the test most often used to measure B_{12} levels, the radiodilution assay method, is shockingly unreliable. In the words of two physicians reporting in the *Journal of the American Medical Association,* the test is "totally ineffective." Kenneth L. Cohen, M.D., and Ronald M. Donaldson, Jr., M.D., both of the Yale University School of Medicine, screened 352 patients using the standard commercial vitamin B_{12} test. None of the patients was revealed by the test to have a B_{12} deficiency. Realizing only too well that they had not uncovered an epidemic of health, the doctors selected 52 persons whose B_{12} measurements were in the lower half of the "normal" range, and were able to get 42 of them to come in for retesting with a combination of other testing methods. Of this group, 36 percent had *abnormally* low vitamin B_{12} levels! Both doctors advise their colleagues to find out

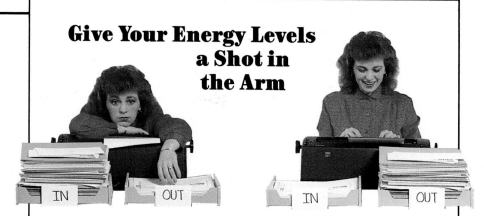

Give Your Energy Levels a Shot in the Arm

"It's Monday!" can't explain why you're pooped before you pop out of bed *every* day of the week.

Maybe instead of looking for an excuse, you should look for an extra boost of B_{12}. There's a reason the nutrient has been touted as a treatment for tiredness: It helps create the healthy red blood cells that transport energy-giving oxygen in the bloodstream.

Robert Donaldson, M.D., professor of medicine at Yale University, explains, "It's well known that many patients receive B_{12} injections because [B_{12}] seems to make them feel better, and it has no adverse side effects."

People who've had stomach or intestinal surgery, as well as other people who simply lack the intrinsic factor necessary to absorb B_{12}, are good candidates for B_{12} injections. They may mean the difference between feeling peppy or pooped.

what kind of test is going to be performed on the blood samples they send out for B_{12} testing. If they find that the commercial kit is being used, they should not rely solely on the test results, but should carefully review all cases of nervous system and mental disturbance, as well as anemia, unless they are *sure* the cause is something other than vitamin B_{12} deficiency.

FOLATE FOR HEALTHY BLOOD

Folate (also called folic acid) is essential to the formation of healthy red blood cells. A severe deficiency over a long enough period can result in megaloblastic anemia, an often fatal and once all-too-common hazard of pregnancy in which the red blood cells enlarge beyond the bloodstream's ability to carry them. For pregnant women, the RDA for folate is double the norm, or 800 micrograms, and nursing mothers need 500 micrograms daily.

Often a folate deficiency will spark anemia and fatigue, and the over-60 group, in particular, should keep a sharp eye out for a possible deficiency, as it has been suggested that one of the curses of the aging process is loss of the ability to absorb folate. While the arguments both for and against this controversial idea are being weighed, there's rather impressive evidence that many senior citizens simply don't ingest enough of the vitamin to stave off anemia.

Research presented at the Florida Symposium on Micronutrients in Human Nutrition at the University of Florida revealed that anemia in the low-income elderly is usually due to a lack of folate and rarely, as is often supposed, due to a lack of iron. The researchers found that 60 percent of the senior citizens tested in Miami had folate levels below normal, although none had an iron deficiency.

Other research from the University of Florida showed that in a large group of Miami teenagers studied, folate levels (and iron levels) were "less than adequate," placing them also at risk for anemia.

Folate has many benefits when used medically; doctors are starting to rely on its curative properties as an alternative to some drugs.

Research at the University of Alabama has shown that folate may be able to arrest or reverse a condition known as cervical dysplasia in women who are on the Pill. Apparently, taking the Pill can cause localized folate deficiencies in the uterus, leading to cervical dysplasia. Left untreated, the condition can progress into cancer.

But folate improves the condition to the point where "supplementation may help reduce the risk of cervical cancer," according to the *Journal of the American Medical Association.*

Nowadays, too, more and more physicians are looking into folate deficiency as a cause of depression. A study at McGill University in Montreal examined the folate levels of three different groups of patients: those who were depressed, those who were psychiatrically ill but not depressed and those who were medically ill.

The researchers discovered that "serum folic acid levels were significantly lower in the depressed patients than in the psychiatric and medical patients . . . . On the basis of our results, we believe that folic acid deficiency depression may exist."

Look for folate in the nearest patch of leafy green vegetables— spinach, beet greens and kale, to name a few. Liver and kidney also provide excellent amounts of the nutrient.

One caution, though: Folate is easily destroyed by cooking, so a careful, quick steaming is in order. A

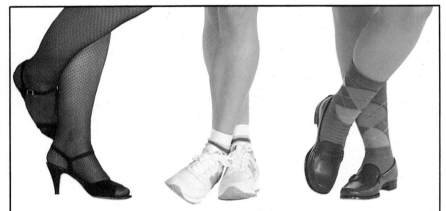

Folate Quiets Restless Legs

Montreal physician M.I. Botez, M.D., is sure there's a connection between lack of folate and a condition known as restless legs syndrome, which afflicts pregnant women. Those who get it complain of creeping, irritating sensations in the lower legs. Dr. Botez points out that restless legs often occur in the last stages of pregnancy, just when folate stores drop lowest. When he and an associate examined 2 groups of pregnant women, they found that 8 of 10 not receiving supplemental folate had the syndrome. But only 1 of 11 taking folate had the problem. When 3 women with severe restless legs syndrome were given 10 milligrams of folate daily, their symptoms vanished after 8 days.

folate supplement might be a good idea if you're in any one of the groups who are prone to a deficiency, such as the elderly or pregnant women.

PANTOTHENATE— THE "ANTISTRESS" VITAMIN

The name pantothenate (or pantothenic acid) comes from the Greek word *pantos,* meaning everywhere—probably because it's found in almost all foods. It's also *needed* everywhere when it comes to producing energy in the body, for pantothenate is what the body uses to build coenzyme A (CoA), a catalyst that converts fats, carbohydrates and proteins into energy.

Not surprisingly, there seems to be a link between pantothenate and fatigue. When levels of CoA fall, the results can be dangerous. In one experiment at the University of Nebraska, Hazel Fox, Ph.D., and colleagues compared two groups of men—one group received the vitamin and the other was totally deprived of it. After ten weeks, the deprived men were listless and complained of fatigue.

That was an extreme case, but Dr. Fox has found that most Americans consume barely as much as the minimum RDA, which ranges from 4 to 7 milligrams. "The intake of pantothenic acid by Americans is decreasing," she says. "In 1955, when I first measured the intake of the vitamin by college women here in Lincoln, the average was about 7 milligrams a day. We rarely get figures that high now. The average is 4 or 5. People just don't eat three square meals the way they used to. People aren't choosing the right foods. There are too many processed foods."

"Fatigue has been described as a symptom of pantothenic acid deficiency," she adds, "and I would make a guarded statement that the evidence shows a relationship between fatigue and low pantothenic acid intake. It's something we need to look into."

There's also evidence that pantothenate is remarkably effective in

The Life-Extension Vitamin

Can pantothenate, a B vitamin, add more years to your life? Since the 1930s, researchers have been exploring the theory that pantothenate somehow slows biochemical processes in the body. And some of the proof that it does comes from Roger Williams, Ph.D., the first man to isolate, identify and synthesize the nutrient. He conducted an experiment with 2 groups of mice, feeding both of them identical and nutritionally complete diets. One group, however, got pantothenate in its drinking water. The animals without added pantothenate lived an average of 550 days. But those getting the extra pantothenate lived an average of 653 days. "If the 550 days is regarded as equivalent to 75 years for a human," Dr. Williams wrote, "then the 653 days would be equivalent to 89 years." He speculated that, "on a purely statistical basis," as much as 10 years can be added to the human life span through supplementation with pantothenate.

relieving hay fever symptoms. The mechanism is not clearly understood, but the testimonies of patients and allergists lend credence to its use as a supplement during the pollen season.

LAST, BUT FAR FROM LEAST

Other vitamins on the B team are biotin, inositol and PABA. Choline, a substance that's technically not a vitamin, is also grouped with the B's. Some of their functions in the body are still not well understood, but thanks to the work of nutritional scientists we know that they all have therapeutic properties.

Take inositol, for instance. As myoinositol (a chemically similar form), it seems to be involved in preventing the nerve damage that often causes pain, numbness and impotence in diabetics. Clinical trials with 15 patients at the Diabetes Hospital in Birmingham, Alabama, conducted by Rex S. Clements, M.D., revealed "a statistically significant improvement in nerve function on the high-myoinositol diet." Not

surprisingly, diabetics excrete much more inositol in the urine than healthy people, which implies an increased need for the nutrient.

Victims of multiple sclerosis (MS) also seem to need more inositol than the general population. According to Viggo Holm, M.D., of Denmark, in people with MS the body's metabolism of inositol may be abnormally rapid.

This could provoke a deficiency of the nutrient, which in turn could lead to destruction of the myelin sheaths protecting the nerves. Dr. Holm found that in 86 normal people and 12 people with MS, none of the former group had abnormal inositol metabolism, but 27 percent of the MS group metabolized inositol "in an abnormally pronounced way."

In addition, inositol has been found helpful in relieving liver problems.

Good food sources include fruits, meat, milk and whole grains. Milling destroys inositol: One slice of enriched white bread contains 6 milligrams, compared to 35.5 milligrams in a slice of whole wheat bread.

PABA Screens the Sun

What with all the reports of sun-induced skin cancer, even mad dogs and Englishmen don't venture out in the noonday sun without first applying a good sunscreen. And the best of the sunscreens out there on the pharmacy shelves contain one of the B vitamins, para-aminobenzoic acid—PABA, for short. Scientists at Harvard Medical School reported that, of 24 screening agents tested, a solution of 5 percent PABA in alcohol provided by far the best protection against ultraviolet radiation. Not only was PABA discovered to be the best sunscreen, but it was found to confine its screening action to that part of the ultraviolet spectrum that causes most of the burning. Less dangerous ultraviolet and visible light that promote tanning got through, while the burning rays were blocked. And tanning without burning, of course, is the whole point of the sunbathing ritual. Since the study at Harvard, improved products have come on the market that outperform the 5 percent PABA solution, but they themselves are based on chemical derivatives of PABA. Apply a sunscreen liberally 45 minutes before going out in the sun to give the active ingredients time to sink in. And remember, all sun preparations wash off easily and should be reapplied every 2 hours or after a swim.

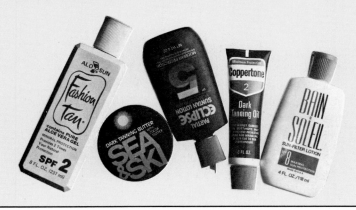

A BETTER MEMORY

Another versatile and therapeutic member of the B family is choline, which is known to prevent lapses of memory and provide relief from some serious nerve disorders.

Researchers agree that the body converts choline into acetylcholine, a chemical necessary for the smooth flow of messages throughout the nervous system. Without acetylcholine, thinking, muscle coordination and other routine functions of the nervous system would be disrupted.

Ronald Mervis, Ph.D., of Ohio State University, thinks that supplemental choline also maintains the "structural integrity of synapses," which are the points of communication between nerve cells in the brain. Because of this, Dr. Mervis believes that supplemental choline may help *prevent* memory loss, and suggests that people get their choline from lecithin, a food supplement that contains the substance. "And we're not talking about a large dose," he adds, "only about 2 tablespoons of lecithin granules per day."

One study, carried out by the National Institute of Mental Health, indicated that a single 10-gram dose of choline can significantly improve memory and recall in normal, healthy people. Interestingly enough, subjects whose memories were poorest at the start of the study were the ones choline helped the most.

But choline may do even more for patients suffering from Alzheimer's disease, a form of mental deterioration that includes severe memory loss.

Also, large oral doses of choline have been used successfully to reduce the involuntary facial twitching of tardive dyskinesia, a disease caused by major tranquilizers like thorazine and common among patients in mental hospitals.

BIOTIN: A BABY'S BLESSING

Biotin deficiency is uncommon. Not only is biotin found in numerous foods, but it is also one of the vitamins synthesized in the body by the action of intestinal bacteria. Most reported cases of deficiency have occurred in people who consume extraordinary amounts of raw egg white, which contains a biotin-binding protein called avidin. But we're talking here about eating over 2 dozen eggs per day!

In recent years, though, doctors have described cases of infants born with biotin dependency, in which requirements for the B vitamin are unusually high. The cause may be malabsorption or an inherited defect in biotin metabolism. A child on an intravenous solution that contains insufficient biotin is also susceptible, as are babies fed biotin-deficient formulas. The symptoms are frighteningly obvious to physicians who know enough to recognize them: The baby suffers from hair loss, inflamed eyes, muscle weakness and a scaly rash (dermatitis). Eventually, he can hardly crawl or sit steadily, and may lose the ability to hold his head upright.

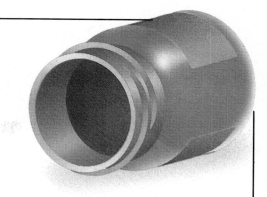

B₁₅: The Vitamin That Isn't

Pangamic acid, also dubbed "vitamin B_{15}," is said to help heart disease, diabetes, alcoholism, asthma, nerve and joint infections, athletic stress—you name it. But "panacea," not pangamic, is what the acid should be called. Studies to date on the substance have been sloppy, and as yet there is no clear chemical identity for it. Most companies making B_{15} call the result calcium pangamate, which contains DMG, an abbreviation for the essential extract that is supposedly so beneficial. But DMG has been shown to be a potential cancer-causing substance, as has DIPA-DCA, which is in some products called B_{15}.

Fortunately, giving biotin to the children reverses those symptoms and sets them on the road to health.

What happens in these cases? It seems that certain enzymes depend on biotin in order to function normally. Without those enzymes, the body can't utilize carbohydrates, proteins and fats. When that happens, specific abnormal metabolites (poisons) build up in the body, creating a whole host of devastating symptoms.

Researchers in Australia and England have uncovered evidence that babies who are victims of sudden infant death syndrome (SIDS) also have lower than normal amounts of biotin and may benefit from supplements of the nutrient.

"We do not suggest," wrote the researchers in *Nature*, "that SIDS results from biotin deficiency alone, but . . . we postulate that biotin insufficiency may leave the infant in a condition in which SIDS can be triggered by mild stress—for example, infection, a missed meal, excessive heat or cold or a changed environment."

5

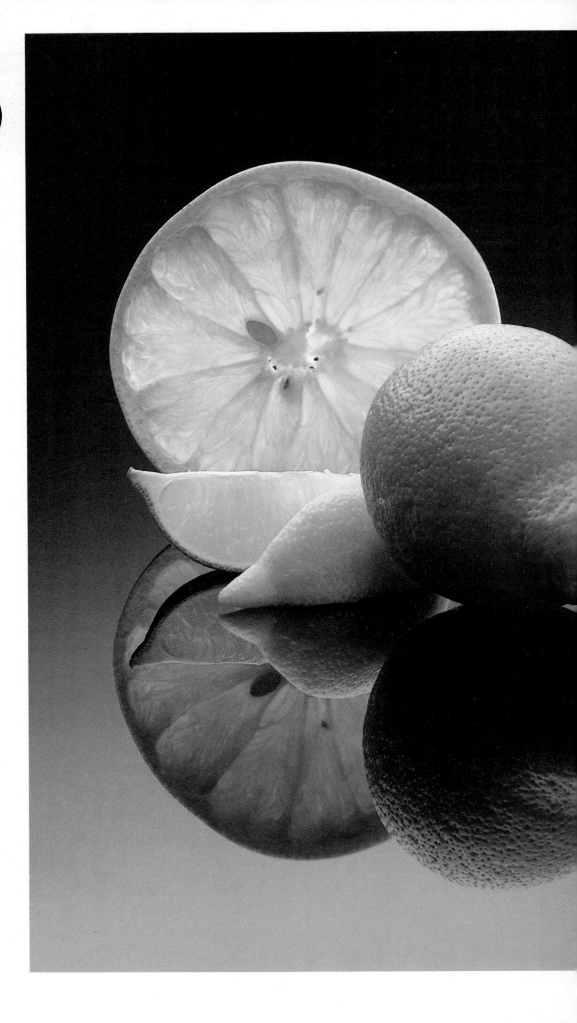

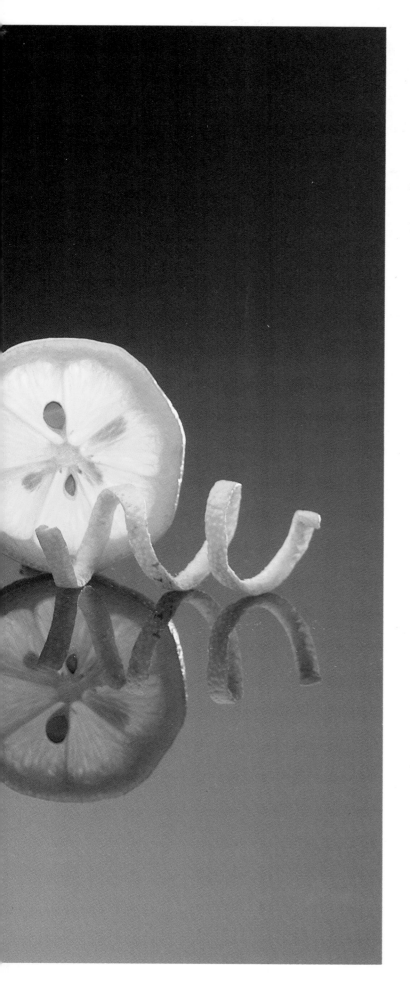

Vitamin C: A Natural Ally

This nutrient has a knack for defending us in tough situations— from colds to cancer.

"Vitamin C is unique among vitamins because it is the only one that seems to play a role in every bodily function, as it holds the cells together," observes Reginald Passmore, M.D., professor of physiology at Edinburgh University in Scotland. "When it is deficient, furthermore, it wreaks more havoc in more places in the body . . . than any other nutrient."

Adds Irwin Stone, D.Sc., one of the early pioneers of vitamin C research: "Ascorbic acid (vitamin C) is involved in so many vital biochemical processes and is so important in daily living that, after 40 years of research, we still have no clear idea of all the ways in which it works."

It's such a versatile performer, in fact, that vitamin C has been called "an oil for the machinery of life." Yet your body can't manufacture it or store more than a few grams, so keeping your cells saturated with a rich, daily supply of C is crucial. Just how crucial it is has been demonstrated in studies showing what happens when you *don't:* Deficiencies interfere with everything from the production of collagen, the protein "cement" that holds your cells together and helps in the healing of wounds, to your ability to digest food and fight the effects of stress.

Researchers at Cornell University have even found that deficiencies impair the body's ability to metabolize drugs, which could have serious implications for the elderly in particular.

"In guinea pigs, we've found that deficiencies of vitamin C impair the liver's ability to detoxify drugs, which results in more of the drug affecting the body—causing, in effect, an overdose," one researcher says.

But what would happen to you if your body tissues were *drenched* with vitamin C, saturated like the soil after a downpour? And what if this soaking lasted not for just a few hours, but for days and days, for the rest of your life?

The fate that would befall you would likely be better health. That's the opinion of a growing number of researchers who are looking into the vitamin C requirements of your body. The word is that the right daily intake of C is the one that ensures this maximum permea-

---

Vitamin C-Rich Recipe: Fruit Cup with Yogurt Sauce

Makes 6 servings

2 cups plain yogurt	2 navel oranges, peeled
6 tablespoons frozen	and sectioned
unsweetened pine-	2 kiwi fruits, peeled and
apple juice	sliced
concentrate,	1 pint strawberries
thawed	

Mix yogurt and pineapple juice concentrate to make a sauce. Combine orange sections, kiwi slices and strawberries. Divide fruit mixture among 6 champagne glasses and spoon sauce over each. Garnish with a strawberry or a kiwi slice.

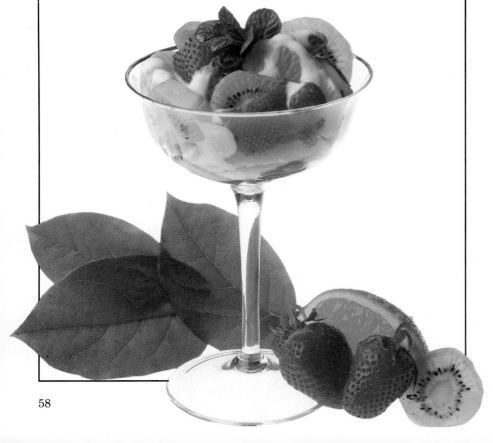

tion of your tissues, a so-called steady state.

It's a condition that exists almost everywhere in the animal world, and that fact set a lot of people thinking about the implications for man. Unlike humans, most animals can synthesize (manufacture) vitamin C internally. Since these C-makers have high saturation levels of the vitamin, scientists reasoned, the steady state must be ideal for their health. Thus, the same saturation condition might be optimum for humans, who have to make sure their C intake keeps their tissues loaded.

Emil Ginter, Ph.D., a distinguished vitamin C researcher from Czechoslovakia, was among the first to test these assumptions. Initially he set out to discover what a maximum saturation of C would do for a creature that shares man's inability to synthesize it—the guinea pig. In test after test he found that guinea pigs on close to maximum saturation levels of C fared better than guinea pigs with lower levels. The animals with higher vitamin C levels handled cholesterol better and developed fewer gallstones when placed on a gallstone-producing diet. The saturation animals not only were better off than those guinea pigs on deficiency intakes of C, but also were even healthier than those getting many times the intake needed to prevent scurvy. (Scurvy is, by dictionary definition, an extreme deficiency of vitamin C resulting in "spongy, swollen and bleeding gums, hemorrhages, and extreme weakness.")

Evidence is accumulating that in humans, too, a state of vitamin C saturation is optimum for health, says Dr. Ginter. Here and abroad, studies have demonstrated that a full store of C can help battle harmful levels of cholesterol and triglycerides (blood fats linked to heart disease), detoxify potentially dangerous histamine (a hormone linked to allergy) and neutralize unwholesome chemicals in your diet.

BEYOND THE RDA

What daily intake will keep your cache of C—your body pool—brimming?

Whatever the quantity is, many researchers and doctors are convinced that it has little to do with the Recommended Dietary Allowance of 60 milligrams a day. "Sixty milligrams is enough, all right—if you want merely to stay just above scurvy level," says W. M. Ringsdorf Jr., D.M.D., of the University of Alabama in Birmingham. "But if you want to live a life of reduced infection, if you want to promote healing and sharpen your immune system, if you want optimum triglyceride levels in your blood, you'll want a daily intake of C far above the RDA," Dr. Ringsdorf adds.

"It is certain," notes Dr. Ginter, "that the officially recommended doses are unable to ensure a maximum body pool, for they do not lead to maximum levels of ascorbate [vitamin C] . . . in the blood, and much less in tissues."

If you examine the C content of human tissues, explains Dr. Ginter, you discover that the maximum pool is actually about 5,000 milligrams (approximately 32 milligrams of C per pound of body weight). And that's similar to the pool values found in monkeys.

"Vitamin C doses necessary for maintaining such a high body pool in humans have not as yet been experimentally determined," Dr. Ginter points out, "but they may be calculated approximately from available data." Since we know the turnover and absorption rate of C, he says, it's a simple matter to compute the intake we need to keep our reservoirs topped off at 5,000 milligrams: about 200 milligrams a day.

That's for the healthy person. Smokers, diabetics, the elderly, people under stress, allergy sufferers and persons taking certain drugs are all in need of extra vitamin C—above and beyond the minimum saturation intake. When your body is under the gun, it demands additional C to heal itself or fight off enemies within.

A diet rich in fresh fruits, vegetables and greens should provide plenty of vitamin C. Steam your vegetables—don't boil them—to retain vitamin C. (The nutrient is water soluble and quickly leaches into cooking water.) And if you take supplements as insurance, you'll gain

The Best Food Sources of Vitamin C

Food	Portion	Vitamin C (mg.)
Orange juice, fresh squeezed	1 cup	124
Green peppers, raw, chopped	½ cup	96
Grapefruit juice, fresh squeezed	1 cup	94
Papaya	½ medium	94
Brussels sprouts	4 sprouts	73
Broccoli, raw, chopped	½ cup	70
Orange	1 medium	70
Cantaloupe	¼ medium	56
Turnip greens, cooked	½ cup	50
Cauliflower, raw, chopped	½ cup	45
Strawberries	½ cup	42
Grapefruit	½ medium	41
Tomato juice	1 cup	39
Potato	1 medium	31
Tomato, raw	1 medium	28
Cabbage, raw, chopped	½ cup	21
Blackberries	½ cup	15
Spinach, raw, chopped	½ cup	14
Blueberries	½ cup	9
Cherries, sweet	½ cup	5
Mung bean sprouts	¼ cup	5

better results taking vitamin C in divided doses throughout the day or in one dose after a meal, according to a study done by researchers from the University of Toronto Faculty of Pharmacy and the University of Arizona College of Pharmacy.

Some people find that vitamin C can cause gassiness or loose stools, a problem quickly corrected by reducing the initial dosage.

Because iron and vitamin C work together, you might also plan to take your supplement of C along with your iron supplement or with iron-rich foods. It's been shown that vitamin C boosts the body's absorption of iron by four times, compared with iron taken alone.

Alcohol, however, works against vitamin C by interfering with absorption. In a study at Deakin University in Victoria, Australia, five healthy volunteers agreed to eat a very odd breakfast: a buttered bun, coffee, 2 grams of vitamin C and 35 grams of ethanol, or ethyl alcohol (roughly equivalent to two martinis or three light beers). Later, they ate a boozeless breakfast for purposes of comparison. Result? "Plasma [blood] ascorbic acid concentrations were significantly lower for at least 24 hours" after the alcoholic meal, wrote the researchers in the *American Journal of Clinical Nutrition.*

VITAMIN C PERKS UP A SAGGING DEFENSE

One of the most important gears the "oil of life" greases is that of the body's immune system—your defense against infectious disease. In one study at South Africa's University of Pretoria, vitamin C was found to stimulate the immune system in two different ways.

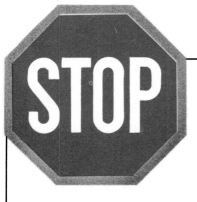

Bladder Infections

Bladder infection? Chronic bladder infection? Well, one answer to that has always been cranberry juice. That could be because it's rich in vitamin C—1 cup has 108 milligrams, just a little less than a cup of fresh-squeezed orange juice. Vitamin C's "presence in the urine may actually promote good health in the bladder and kidneys," says Alan Gaby, M.D., of Baltimore, Maryland. Rather than inhibiting bacterial growth by acidifying the urine, Dr. Gaby says, "It can kill some bacteria, including *E. coli,* the most common cause of urinary tract infections." Cranberry juice also works because it contains hippuric acid, which inhibits the growth of bacteria. One doctor reported in a medical journal that he has used cranberry juice in his practice for 20 years, and that it consistently clears up bladder infections. He recommends a 6-ounce glass twice daily for continued relief of symptoms.

When a germ, virus or any other microscopic invader penetrates the body's first line of defense, a healthy immune system musters an army of defenders and hustles them off to the site of the invasion. One division of this defending army is made up of specialized white blood cells called neutrophils, which simply eat up the enemy. In both human subjects and human cells in test tubes, the South African scientists found that vitamin C increased the mobility of these neutrophils, speeding up their migration to the front lines.

How do neutrophils know where the attackers have broken through the front lines and how to get to the scene of the invasion? They do it by following the "scent" of a chemical distress signal the body produces when it becomes inflamed by injury. The neutrophils' amazing journey through the body's byways, hard on the enemy's trail like a brace of police bloodhounds, is called "chemotaxis"—and it doesn't always work. When neutrophils are exposed to a chemotactic signal once, they become deactivated—that is, they fail to respond to a subsequent signal.

Yet Italian researchers have found that vitamin C "completely prevented the loss of true chemotactic responsiveness by cells." In other words, human neutrophils, exposed to a chemical distress signal, responded right on cue to a second signal—*if* they were saturated with vitamin C. Otherwise, they didn't respond at all.

Vitamin C also helps stimulate the immune response by stepping up the body's production of lymphocytes, another kind of white blood cell.

These two processes are at the heart of the immune system's effectiveness, which means that vitamin C should help fight *many* types of infection. And it does. Benjamin V. Siegel, Ph.D., and Brian Leibovitz, researchers at the University of Oregon Health Sciences Center in Portland, noted in the *International Journal of Vitamin and Nutrition Research* that vitamin C has been demonstrated effective in humans against hepatitis, measles, mumps, cold sores, meningitis and other viruses, as well as bacterial and fungal disease agents. "It appears that ascorbic acid may play an important role in the immune response," they concluded.

In his research, Dr. Siegel has found that mice treated with large doses of vitamin C are better able to resist leukemia virus than untreated animals. In fact, the vitamin C group was able to manufacture 100 percent more interferon, a protein produced inside the body that can inhibit virus multiplication.

On a weight basis, the mice in Dr. Siegel's study received the equivalent of 15 grams of vitamin C daily for a 150-pound man.

But what about something a little milder, like the common cold?

AN UNCOMMONLY GOOD TREATMENT FOR THE COMMON COLD

Whether or not vitamin C has a significant effect on the all-too-common cold has been a matter of scientific debate for years. Because the results of studies have varied so widely, it has been suggested that different people may metabolize the vitamin in widely different ways. But nonetheless, study after study has shown that people who take vitamin C have fewer and milder colds.

In an Australian study, for instance, 95 pairs of identical twins—perfectly matched for age, sex and genetic makeup—were used to compare the cold-fighting power of vitamin C with that of a placebo. For 100 days, one of each pair of twins took a gram (1,000 milligrams) of vitamin C daily while the other took the placebo, though neither knew which was which. They were also asked to make careful note of the duration and severity of colds, should they appear.

When the results were analyzed, the research team concluded that vitamin C was responsible for shortening the average duration of cold episodes by 19 percent.

In a study at the University of Toronto, 407 people received 1,000 milligrams of vitamin C a day and an extra 3,000 milligrams a day for the first three days of a cold. Another 411 people received a worthless

A Natural Antihistamine

The symptoms of nasal allergy—the runny nose, its inflamed and swollen lining—are produced when histamine reacts with allergens. Histamine is a chemical naturally produced by the body. And when it meets up with dust or pollen—bang!—your nose is off and running. But relief can be found with vitamin C, because it's a natural *anti*histamine.

Researchers had 17 volunteers inhale histamine and measured their levels of "airway constriction." The next day, the volunteers again received histamine—but this time they also got 500 milligrams of vitamin C. The degree of constriction was much less.

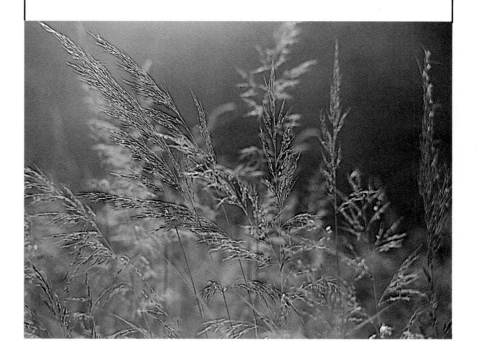

placebo. Compared with the placebo group, the vitamin C group spent 30 percent fewer days indoors because of illness and missed 33 percent fewer days of work, according to the *Canadian Medical Association Journal.*

In a study of crew members on a Polaris submarine, 37 sailors who received 2,000 milligrams of vitamin C a day had 66 percent fewer cold symptoms than a placebo group.

In a government study of soldiers undergoing training in northern Canada, those receiving 1,000 milligrams of vitamin C a day had about 68 percent less illness than a placebo group.

And in another study from Toronto, 448 people who took vitamin C had up to 38 percent fewer cold symptoms—runny nose, fever, sore throat, tight chest, aching limbs and depression—than a placebo group.

Vitamin C Aces Fatigue

Vitamin C may play a crucial role in maintaining our energy supply. Experiments with animals have shown that an increase in vitamin C increases the amount of glycogen stored in muscles and the liver—a crucial fact because glycogen is our energy-storage material. Researchers have also conducted experiments on people to see if supplementation with vitamin C "increases resistance to fatigue and [promotes] increased work output."

For instance, Emanuel Cheraskin, M.D., D.M.D., professor and chairman of the department of oral medicine, University of Alabama Medical Center, Birmingham, surveyed over 400 people. He rated them according to their symptoms of fatigue and intake of vitamin C. The fatigue "score" of the 330 people who consumed more than 400 milligrams of vitamin C daily was *half* that of the 81 people who took less than 100 milligrams daily.

What's more, researchers have found that vitamin C may make you more alert. A study of a group of coal miners found that those miners taking C suffered far fewer accidental injuries than those who didn't receive supplements.

"There is little doubt," wrote the authors of the Toronto study in the *Canadian Medical Association Journal,* "that the intake of additional vitamin C can lead to a reduced burden of winter illness."

THE TAMING OF THE FLU

Fortunately, vitamin C's protective benefits seem to extend to the flu virus as well. As biochemist and Nobel laureate Linus Pauling, Ph.D., says, "The common cold is a nuisance, but is not very dangerous. Only rarely does it lead to complications that cause death. Influenza (the flu), on the other hand, is a very serious and dangerous disease. In the great influenza pandemic of 1918-1919 the disease was contracted by about 85 percent of the population in all countries and [it] killed about 1 percent. . . ."

He continues, "The best protection against the flu is one's natural defense mechanisms. These defense mechanisms seem to have protected about one-sixth of the people during the 1918-1919 pandemic, presumably for the most part those people whose defense mechanisms were operating most effectively. There is much evidence . . . that a good intake of vitamin C improves the functioning of the natural defense mechanisms to such an extent that a much larger fraction of the population would resist the infection."

The miseries associated with hay fever and certain allergies are very similar to those of the common cold and flu. Vitamin C is helpful for these conditions, too, because it is a natural antihistamine.

In a series of studies, researchers from the department of obstetrics and gynecology at Methodist Hospital in Brooklyn found that blood levels of vitamin C bore an inverse relationship to blood levels of histamine; if C levels went up, histamine levels went down, and vice versa.

In one instance, the researchers took 11 people with low levels of vitamin C (high levels of histamine) and placed them on a program of vitamin C supplementation. Improvement was rapid.

A SHIELD AGAINST STRESS

Let's say you're flat on your back in the hospital, recovering from abdominal surgery. Or money problems are weighing on your mind. Or you're walking down a city street, choking on smog. How much vitamin C does your body need now?

More than you might think. "Stress is just one factor that steps up your vitamin C requirements," says Robert Haskell, M.D., of San Francisco. "If anything helps you battle the effects of stress, it's extra vitamin C."

"It appears that all forms of pollution increase the requirements for vitamin C in humans and experimental animals," notes Dr. Emil Ginter. "It has been repeatedly shown that various pesticides, industrial toxins, certain drugs (particularly antipregnancy pills) and smoking decrease blood vitamin C levels."

From mental pressure to environmental toxins, we can lessen the stressful effects (and gain more energy while we're at it) by keeping our bodies and brains well supplied with vitamin C.

As a natural detoxicant, vitamin C may help cleanse the body of ozone—a highly toxic pollutant gas and a major agent in the formation of smog—according to researchers at the University of Queensland in Australia. They exposed mice to various concentrations of ozone in the air for 30 minutes. As much as 50 percent of the vitamin C in their lung tissue was lost during that time. The vitamin seemed to be used up in its effort to battle the ozone, say the researchers. Previously, scientists had established that vitamin C can prevent lung damage caused by ozone, but the Australian study strongly supported the conclusion that it was the vitamin C *in the lung itself* that was the preventive.

Other experiments have demonstrated vitamin C's possible protective action against PCBs, the most widespread chemical pollutants in the United States.

In one representative trial published in *Nutrition Reports International*, researchers fed young laboratory animals high doses of the

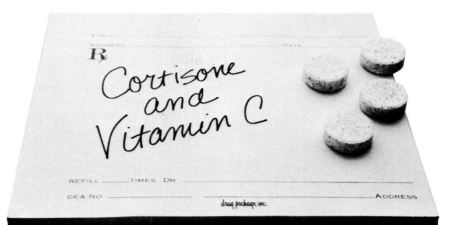

You don't have to look very far to find someone taking one of the steroid drugs—cortisone, hydrocortisone, prednisone or a related compound—despite their many undesirable side effects. That's why it's encouraging to learn that vitamin C can counteract some of them.

One of the most dangerous consequences of steroids is reduced resistance to infection. Steroids interfere with the ability of special corpuscles in the blood to destroy invading bacteria. But extra vitamin C, taken at the same time as the drug, can restore this natural defense mechanism, according to scientists at the University of Louisville School of Medicine. They concluded that for patients receiving certain steroids, "ascorbic acid may be beneficial in reducing the high incidence of infection."

chemicals. The animals grew poorly and developed high levels of cholesterol. (PCBs are known to interfere with fat metabolism.) The animals also excreted *44 times* more vitamin C in their urine—a sign, according to the researchers, that the animals' bodies were synthesizing large quantities of the vitamin in an attempt to detoxify PCBs.

Next, the researchers fed another group of animals PCBs—but also gave them vitamin C to see if it would help protect them against the pollutant. These animals grew normally and had normal cholesterol levels. They also had a "normal outward appearance," compared to the sickly appearance of the PCB animals who didn't get vitamin C.

THE NUTRIENT THAT MAY THWART CANCER

"It is now widely accepted that ascorbic acid nutritional status markedly affects the toxicity and/or carcinogenicity of greater than 50 pollutants, many of which are ubiquitous in the air, water and food environments," says Edward J. Calabrese, Ph.D., associate professor of environmental health at the University of Massachusetts in Amherst.

In other words, the vitamin is proven to detoxify the very agents that can expose our bodies to cancer. And that's especially true of nitrosa-

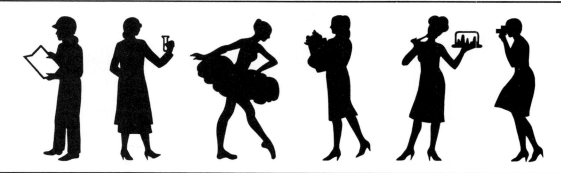

Ladies' Choice for Cancer Protection

When a cure for cancer is finally discovered, chances are that it will have a lot to do with nutrition, according to W. Robert Bruce, M.D., Ph.D., of the Ludwig Institute in Toronto. Much of Dr. Bruce's research has centered on vitamin C therapy for prevention of malignancies of the breast and uterus. Not long ago, he discovered that supplements of vitamins C and E could help decrease certain substances suspected of promoting cancer of the colon.

Curiously, Dr. Bruce has found that many of the same factors that promote colon cancer are present in breast cancer.

And from Japan, there is more good news.

"Vitamin C is especially effective for cancer of the uterus," a team of Japanese researchers concluded after a 5-year study of terminally ill cancer patients. They found that patients with uterine cancer responded to vitamin C therapy better than those with other forms of cancer.

The life expectancy of women with uterine cancer who received between 5 and 30 grams of vitamin C daily was more than 15 times that of women who received only 4 grams or less per day. (These amounts should be used only under a doctor's supervision.)

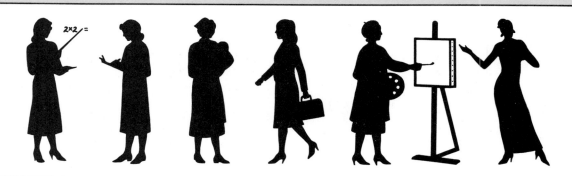

Vitamin C Gives Cancer Patients a Longer Life

Average Survival Time with and without Vitamin C

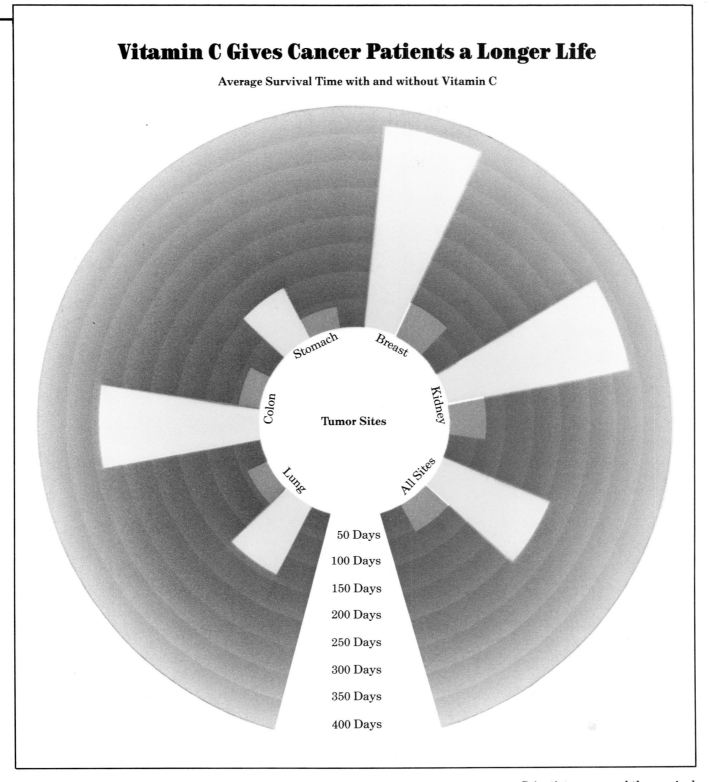

Tumor Sites

Stomach

Breast

Colon

Kidney

Lung

All Sites

50 Days
100 Days
150 Days
200 Days
250 Days
300 Days
350 Days
400 Days

mine formation in the stomach. Nitrosamines are carcinogens (cancer-causing agents) that may be formed when we eat foods treated with sodium nitrate. (Nitrates are added to many processed meat and smoked fish products as preservatives and as flavoring and coloring agents.)

But now evidence suggests that vitamin C can actually prevent the

formation of nitrosamines in your stomach, says Dr. Calabrese. It's a natural detoxifying agent, but only if the vitamin is in your stomach at the same time as the nitrate-treated foods. The obvious solution—taking your vitamin C several times during the day with your meals—is practical for more reasons than one.

"Even if you don't eat foods rich

Scientists compared the survival time of 100 terminal cancer patients given vitamin C with 1,000 similar patients who did not receive the vitamin. They found that "the administration of [vitamin C] . . . to patients with advanced cancer leads to about a fourfold increase in their life expectancy. . . ."

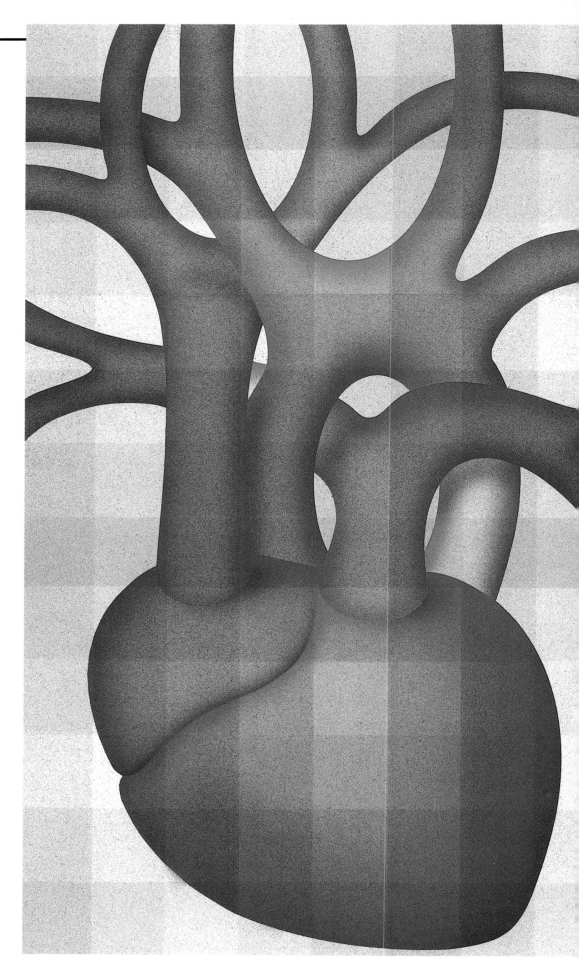

How can you keep your heart the picture of health? With vitamin C. It may help lower cholesterol, keep the blood cells from forming an artery-clogging clot and prevent the formation of plaque, circulatory debris that can stop the flow of life-giving oxygen to the heart.

in nitrates, you are still exposed to those chemicals," says Steven R. Tannenbaum, Ph.D., professor of toxicology and food chemistry at Massachusetts Institute of Technology. "That's because your body manufactures them automatically. Eating cured foods only adds to the level that's already there."

Other researchers, such as Dr. Pauling and Dr. Ewan Cameron of Scotland, also believe that vitamin C significantly reduces our chances of succumbing to cancer.

"My present estimate," Dr. Pauling says, "is that the incidence and mortality from cancer could be decreased by 75 percent by the proper use of vitamin C alone, starting out with taking vitamin C prophylactically. I'm not saying that *will* happen. It will be impossible to get the proper use by everybody. Some people won't take vitamin C every day. Nevertheless, that's what I think would happen if vitamin C were used properly."

Dr. Cameron agrees. "For one thing, several studies have found that cancer patients are almost invariably severely depleted of vitamin C. Several studies throughout the world have found that gastric cancer, for instance, seems to be associated with a lower intake of vitamin C in the diet. Similar studies have shown the same thing with other forms of cancer, such as esophageal cancer, colorectal cancer, bladder cancer. Vitamin C has also been demonstrated to help cancer patients tolerate radiation therapy, *and* improve the therapeutic effect of the radiation."

Scientists around the world continue to examine vitamin C's effects on already-existing cancer cells very closely. In a study at the University of Kansas Medical Center, researchers found that vitamin C suppressed the growth of certain leukemia cells. Interestingly, lower concentrations of vitamin C worked as well as extremely high levels of the vitamin in that particular instance.

Apparently vitamin C also lashes out at certain bad cells while leaving good cells unharmed. A group of researchers from France and the United States found that vitamin C is selectively toxic to at least one type of malignant cell—a melanoma cell.

The researchers extracted both cancerous and noncancerous cells from mice. Then they placed the cells in two separate cultures and added vitamin C. The melanotic (malignant) cells showed a 50 percent decrease in colony formation, cell number and their ability to stay alive.

"Vitamin C may directly inhibit the growth of proliferating cells, and this might explain some of the reported carcinostatic [cancer-suppressing] effects," the researchers reported.

'C' IS FOR CHOLESTEROL— AND ITS CONTROL

Mention cholesterol, and most people want to do something about it. So they start thinking about breakfast. Now, that's not a bad place to start, but they immediately implicate eggs. And that's a crime. What they should be doing is pouring themselves another glass of orange juice. Vitamin C, researchers have found, is a good defense against cholesterol, hardened arteries and heart disease.

One testimony comes from England, where 11 elderly hospital patients with coronary artery problems took 1 gram (1,000 milligrams) of vitamin C daily—resulting in a decrease of total blood cholesterol levels in only six weeks. That prompted researchers, writing in the *Journal of Human Nutrition,* to assert that "atherosclerosis and ischemic heart disease are not inevitable features of aging."

To give a little background on the case, cholesterol's guilt is purely by association. Left to itself, cholesterol actually does some good. It helps our digestion by producing bile, without which we can suffer from gallstones. Our bodies need cholesterol to manufacture vitamin D, and there is some evidence that it protects us from cancer. Its home turf is the liver, but cholesterol goes out a lot. Its traveling companions are called lipoproteins, and they chauffeur it around the bloodstream.

In the company of high-density

lipoproteins (HDL), cholesterol's joyride is relatively safe. But introduce it to low-density lipoproteins (LDL), and look out: Cholesterol is up to no good. Scientists now believe that lowering total cholesterol is less

important than getting most of it on the HDL route. And that, the British research team learned, is another thing vitamin C does.

When they started their gram-a-day supplementation, most of the heart patients had vitamin C deficiencies; the *men* also had correspondingly low levels of HDL cholesterol. "After six weeks' treatment with ascorbic acid, the mean [average] HDL cholesterol concentration had increased," the study noted. What's more, that benefit was not

Keep Your Back Sailing Along

One especially important nutrient in the prevention and treatment of back pain, according to James Greenwood, Jr., M.D., a clinical professor of neurosurgery at the Methodist Hospital in Houston, Texas, is vitamin C.

"Vitamin C's most dramatic effect in my practice these days," says the neurosurgeon,

"is to prevent and relieve muscle soreness resulting from exercise." He also sees "a significant percentage of patients with early spinal disk problems who are able to *avoid surgery* by the use of large doses of vitamin C."

Whether the problem stems from muscles or disks, Dr. Greenwood starts all his patients out on at least 500 milligrams of vitamin C taken with each meal.

restricted to the heart patients; all 7 men in the 14-member healthy control group enjoyed it as well.

The seven women who acted as controls experienced no significant change in lipoprotein cholesterol, but that doesn't mean vitamin C is guilty of sex discrimination. Women naturally have higher HDL levels, which is one reason they are less prone to heart attacks than men. All the women in the control group had healthier HDL levels.

The evidence that vitamin C can protect as well as defend, that it is as beneficial to high-risk subjects as to those already afflicted with heart disease, may be the most compelling aspect of the British investigation. The research team entered a plea for higher recommended daily intake of vitamin C because "latent ascorbic acid deficiency may be one of several preventable 'risk' factors contributing to the present epidemic of ischemic heart disease in the western world."

But vitamin C isn't just a policeman directing cholesterol traffic through the bloodstream and forcing loitering platelets to break it up and move on. After a heart attack has occurred, a high level of C can pay off like an insurance policy.

That's what Scottish physicians at Southern General Hospital in Glasgow reported when they discovered that blood levels of vitamin C drop down to scurvy levels within 6 to 12 hours after a person suffers a heart attack.

They concluded that the vitamin C is diverted to the heart to help rebuild the damaged coronary tissue.

Their findings were supported by a later study in which Jairo Ramirez, M.D., and colleagues at the University of Louisville, Kentucky, found that concentrations of vitamin C in the white blood cells of 150 patients with heart disease were "significantly lower" than those of a control group. And they remained dangerously low for several weeks after a heart attack, before gradually increasing to a stable level.

Dr. Ramirez, now engaged in private practice in San Antonio, Texas, also noted that cholesterol is higher in patients deprived of vitamin C.

As research continues, scientists are finding that the RDA set for vitamin C is seldom enough to guarantee a healthy heart and that wholesome foods we've enjoyed for centuries—such as eggs—are probably not to blame for coronary catastrophes.

One of the first to recognize that fact was England's Dr. Constance Spittle Leslie, who put herself on a high-cholesterol diet, but found that her blood cholesterol *dropped* because she ate lots of fresh fruits and vegetables rich in vitamin C.

If she cooked the fruits and vegetables, however, her blood cholesterol rose, because heat destroys vitamin C. The results were the same when Dr. Leslie carried out the experiment on 58 human volunteers.

She also found that when they were given 1-gram supplements of vitamin C every day, the volunteers enjoyed the drop in cholesterol levels even if they cooked their fruits and vegetables.

THE "MISSION IMPOSSIBLE" VITAMIN

They ought to call vitamin C the "Mission Impossible" vitamin. When an illness looks hopeless or resistant to drugs, it seems, doctors and patients often call for vitamin C as a last resort. Puzzling viral diseases: Try vitamin C. Chronic skin diseases: Try vitamin C.

Vitamin C doesn't work miracles, of course, especially if it arrives late in the course of a disease. But it's amazing how often it does work in certain hospital or laboratory situations that confound doctors and where other therapies have failed or caused prohibitive side effects.

Journalist Norman Cousins, for instance, recovered from an "untreatable" connective tissue disease by taking lots of vitamin C. A friend of Cousins brought his daughter back from viral encephalitis with ice cream loaded with vitamin C. The list goes on, and unexpected applications for vitamin C are being discovered all the time. For example:

Burns and Bedsores. At the Human Tissue Reconstruction Institute at

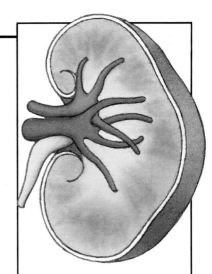

The Stone Truth

The sweeping statement is often made that high doses of vitamin C create the danger of kidney stones. That's true for people with diseased kidneys, but it's not a problem for those with normal kidney function, writes a physician in the *New England Journal of Medicine.* After examining a young man taking 15 grams of vitamin C daily for over 4 months, he said patients with "normal [kidney] function can tolerate exceptionally high doses of this vitamin."

Bethany Methodist Hospital in Chicago, Anthony N. Silvetti, M.D., was confronted with about 30 patients with stubborn bedsores, skin ulcers due to varicose veins or diabetes and burns due to heat or caustic chemicals. These sores had festered for between two months and several *years* with no response to conventional treatments, according to Dr. Silvetti.

Vitamin C helped heal the sores dramatically. Dr. Silvetti prepared a solution of simple and complex sugars along with essential amino acids and vitamin C. He cleared dead tissue from the sores, washed them with a salt solution, then applied his therapeutic mixture every day and covered the sores with sterile, nonadhesive dressings.

"Within the first 24 to 73 hours of beginning the nutrient treatment," Dr. Silvetti and his co-workers reported, "the wounds became cleaner. The foul smell disappeared and the wounds exuded less pus. The infected tissue rapidly transformed into healthy growing tissue full of new blood vessels . . . . Small to medium-sized wounds eventually healed completely with little scarring. Larger wounds accepted early, successful skin grafts."

Skin Health. At the University of Genoa Medical School in Italy, researchers treated patients who were unable to resist bacteria infections normally. Their white blood cells couldn't "chase" or kill bacteria and, as a result, they suffered chronically from abscesses and boils. One patient had had 43 abscesses in two years. None had gone infection free for as long as a year.

Again, vitamin C proved effective without causing side effects. Three of the patients took 1 to 2 grams a day and improved within a few weeks. After a year, their skin was still clear. It was the longest stretch of skin health they had ever enjoyed.

Infertility. In an issue of *Fertility and Sterility,* Earl B. Dawson, Ph.D., of the University of Texas Medical Branch in Galveston, reported the results of a vitamin C preparation (which also contained calcium, magnesium and manganese) on 20 men who were considered infertile due to spermagglutination. (In sperm-agglutination, the sperm clump together and cannot swim normally.) Seven men with the same condition were used as controls, and took no vitamin C.

After 60 days, the wives of all 20 men taking the vitamin C — 1 gram daily — had become pregnant. The 7 men not taking vitamin C remained infertile. The nutrient not only reversed the sperm-clumping condition, it also *raised* sperm counts by 54 percent.

In a later study by Dr. Dawson with 35 infertile men with sperm problems, results with 1 gram of vitamin C daily were seen after just one week. Sperm motility (the ability of sperm to move in a forward motion), viability and total numbers were greatly improved. In fact, the sperm defect was judged to have regressed to the point that fertility

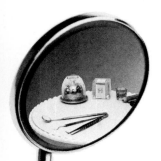

Vitamin C, By Gum!

Experiments have shown that vitamin C might be able to reverse the kind of breakdown seen in gum disease. Researchers looked at samples of cells taken from the gums of 21 volunteers whose diets contained very little vitamin C. Under an electron microscope, the researchers saw the biological equivalent of a tumbled-down brick wall. Collagen and other structural components, which are the bricks and mortar of healthy tissue, were literally broken and disheveled.

But after the volunteers were given 70 milligrams of vitamin C daily for 6 weeks, the cells pulled themselves together and began to look organized and vigorous. The changes "correspond to a very early phase in tissue regeneration," said the researchers. They noted that vitamin C is necessary for the formation of collagen, which is a protein, and that collagen is a critical building block for the gums and a lot of other tissues. Vitamin C deficiency alone won't cause periodontal (gum) disease, the researchers said, but it can make it worse.

was restored after only four days on the supplement.

Polyps. Doctors from West Virginia University gave high doses of vitamin C to nine people to test the vitamin's effect on rectal polyps. (Rectal polyps often lead to rectal cancer.) After from three to seven months of treatment with 3,000 milligrams per day of vitamin C, rectal polyps disappeared in two people and were reduced in three others. Among the other four people, one was unaffected by the vitamin C and the other three stopped taking it.

Rheumatoid Arthritis. A Canadian research team cultured normal and arthritic cells taken from human joints with aspirin, vitamin C, vitamin E and combinations of the three. Aspirin was found to be slightly effective in inhibiting arthritic cell growth and reducing cell population, but "high and low concentrations of vitamin C had little effect on normal cells, and a low concentration had little effect on [arthritic] cells. *However, a high concentration eradicated these [arthritic] cells*" (italics ours), according to the journal *Experientia.*

The researchers concluded that an aspirin-vitamin C combination might be the best way to reduce the growth of arthritic cells.

BIOFLAVONOIDS: PARTNERS IN HEALTH

The effects of the bioflavonoids were first observed in 1936 by scientists led by Nobel laureate Albert Szent-Györgyi. Dr. Szent-Györgyi, who also discovered vitamin C, noted that when animals with scurvy were given crude preparations of vitamin C derived from natural sources, they lived longer than animals given pure vitamin C. The impure vitamin C was more effective in healing the capillary damage that is characteristic of scurvy. Dr. Szent-Györgyi reasoned that there must have been some additional substance present in the impure vitamin C that boosted its healing effects.

That substance was actually a group of compounds, the bioflavonoids. (Bioflavonoids are found, as is

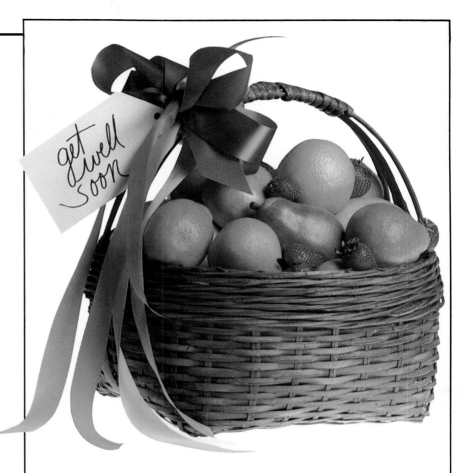

C for Surgery: Before and After

Prepare for surgery by getting enough vitamin C, because the most important link in the healing chain of events is the formation of collagen, which makes healing possible. And there's a good chance of getting too little C during hospitalization, because after any serious injury—surgical wounds included—the body's metabolism of protein and water-soluble vitamins gets jolted into high gear. You can quickly start needing a lot more C than you have.

A vitamin C deficiency can also let you go further "down" under the anesthetic than either you or your surgeon is counting on.

vitamin C, in fresh vegetables and fruits, particularly citrus.) Dr. Szent-Györgyi and his colleagues found that these compounds act to strengthen the capillaries and stop capillary bleeding by lowering the permeability of the capillary walls. These minuscule blood vessels are the link in the circulatory system joining the arteries and the veins. They help carry out the chief function of the circulatory system—they deliver oxygen and nutrients to the body's tissues and remove poisonous wastes.

"The important role which capillary dysfunction plays in many diseases is fully recognized by the medical profession, for it is in the capillary system that the essential exchange of body fluids takes place," a team of American scientists told an International Congress of Physiology.

In a paper delivered to the 20th International Congress of Physiology in Brussels, Belgium, Boris Sokoloff, M.D., William Coda Martin, M.D., and Clarence Saelhof, M.D., listed a variety of diseases in which failure of the capillaries to function properly was a problem. "In viral hepatitis, poliomyelitis, smallpox, measles, primary atypical pneumonia, mumps, virus A influenza, St. Louis encephalitis and other viral infections, capillary fragility and hemorrhage have been observed." The scientists also reported that capillary problems were a factor in arteriosclerosis, hypertension, rheumatoid arthritis, diabetes and bleeding ulcers.

The paper described the researchers' use of bioflavonoids to treat a number of these disorders, particularly those that are likely to strike older people. Age itself tends to produce capillary problems. Tests of 189 patients aged 53 to 88 found that 124 of them, about 64 percent, suffered from capillary fragility. Patients in the group who had high blood pressure were more likely to have capillary problems than those who did not.

The researchers treated 30 of these patients, including 19 suffering from high blood pressure, with bioflavonoids for a period of four weeks. In only one instance was there no change in the patient's condition. In 2 cases there was some improvement, and in the remaining 27 the functioning of the capillaries was either completely or very nearly restored to normal.

The major trauma of miscarriage, too, may be avoidable with bioflavonoid therapy.

"I believe some miscarriages occur because of increased fragility of placental capillaries, and bioflavonoid supplements seem to help toughen those capillaries," says Jack C. Redman, M.D., a family practitioner in Albuquerque, New Mexico. He prescribes citrus bioflavonoids for his patients who suffer from chronic miscarriages. Dr. Redman says his results with the bioflavonoid therapy have been excellent.

"I've had success giving bioflavonoids to women who have had two, three, even four miscarriages," Dr. Redman explains. "I tell them to begin taking the supplements immediately the next time they become pregnant, and it almost always works. My results have been very encouraging."

Hemorrhoids are another problem involving the capillaries. Many doctors advise that bran should be added to the diet of a person suffering from hemorrhoids, because by softening the stool, the bran saves the irritated tissues of a hemorrhoid from more wear and tear. But bran is only a first step. Bioflavonoids could be the second.

One doctor from Switzerland, writing in the *Medical Tribune,* says he has treated over 200 hemorrhoid patients with bioflavonoid therapy. The results, he says, were "extremely encouraging, especially where early stages of the [disease] are concerned . . . . Pain and pruritis [itching] . . . disappeared entirely."

AN END TO EASY BRUISING

Yet another capillary-related condition—bruising—can indicate a need for more bioflavonoids. Frank W. Barr, M.D., of Charlotte, North Carolina, turns to the bioflavonoids first whenever he has patients who are 'easy bruisers.' "I immediately start them on a course of bioflavonoids," he says, "and almost universally get good results after three months."

Bioflavonoids have been found effective in countering several of the complications of diabetes. In diabetes, and also in cases of high blood pressure, inflammation of the retina is a frequent problem. The retina is located at the back of the eyeball, where the images we see are received and carried to the brain by the optic nerve. Inflammation of the retina results in impaired vision, and is accompanied by the buildup of waxy excretions from the blood vessels. One-sixth of all cases of acquired blindness are the result of retinal disease in diabetes.

Dr. Sokoloff and his colleagues found that in 85 percent of 198 cases of retinal inflammation treated with bioflavonoids, the bleeding in the retina was promptly controlled.

Heal Cold Sores in Half the Time!

Bioflavonoids and vitamin C can help your body heal cold sores in half the time usually required, according to researchers at the National Naval Dental Center in Bethesda, Maryland. The painful blisters that erupt in the mouth and around the lips are the result of infection by the herpes simplex virus (Type I). Between 80 and 90 percent of us get them at some time in our lives, and about 40 percent have the problem over and over again.

Commander Geza T. Terezhalmy, D.D.S., the director of the study, reasoned that herpes gets a hold only when tiny blood vessels in the tissue have been damaged. And so he set out to find if the tissue-strengthening ability of bioflavonoids and vitamin C would help protect the lips and mouth from infection.

To do it, he studied 50 cases of recurrent herpes infections. He treated 20 with 600 milligrams each of bioflavonoids and vitamin C divided into 3 daily doses. Twenty were treated with 1,000 milligrams each of bioflavonoids and vitamin C divided into 5 daily doses. And the other 10 got some dummy pills. The results? People treated with the dummy pills were symptom free after an average of 9.7 days. But all of those treated with bioflavonoids and vitamin C were symptom free after only 4.2 days. (For a natural source of bioflavonoids, eat the white core of green peppers along with the rest of the vegetable.)

6

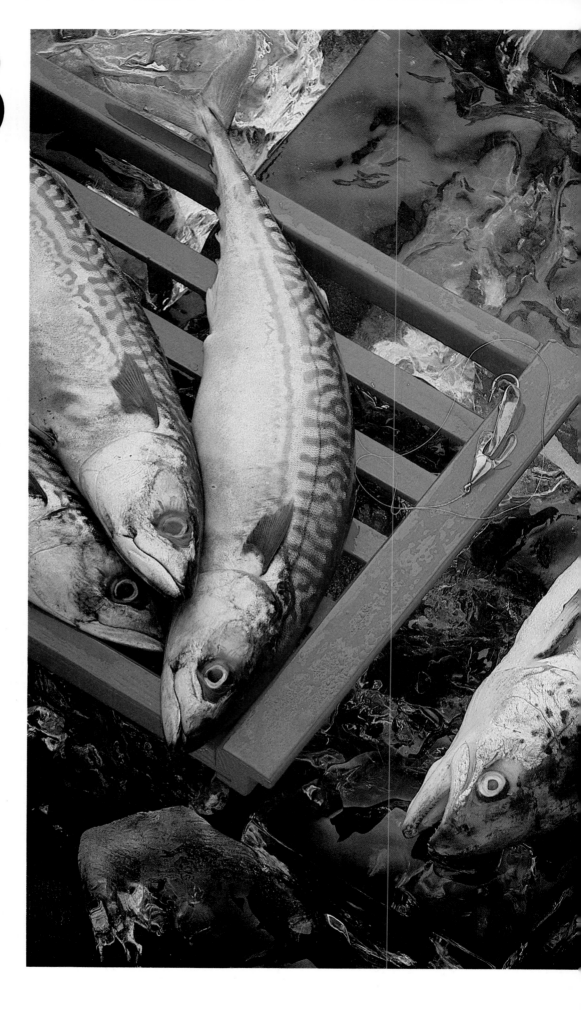

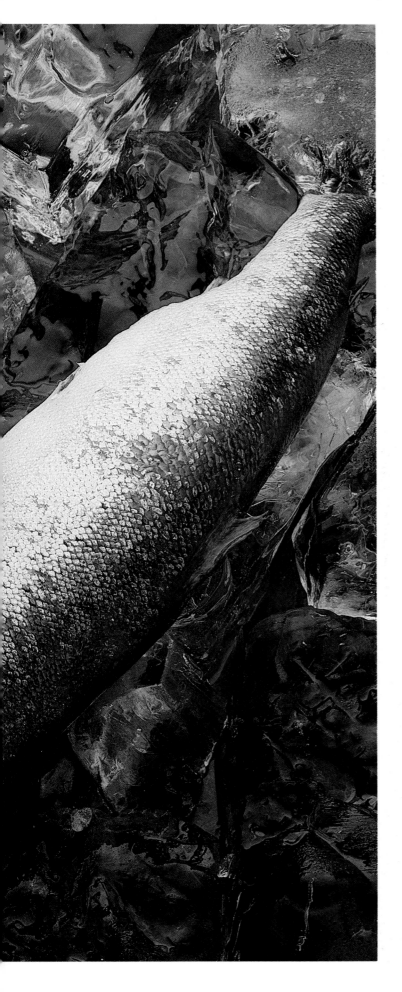

Vitamin D Lets the Sun Shine In

This crucial vitamin strengthens your bones and nourishes your muscles and nerves.

How can the sun affect bone growth? It does so through vitamin D, a remarkable substance that is synthesized when your skin is struck by ultraviolet light. Although vitamin D is available in some foods (see page 77), most of the vitamin D that we use in our bodies comes from the magical meeting of skin and sun.

Vitamin D is unique in that it acts very much like a hormone. It is an activator, prodding calcium and phosphorus into the bloodstream so they can spread their good deeds around. In fact, those two minerals are all-important—not only are they the main ingredients of healthy bones, but they also maintain nerves and muscles.

If your intake or production of vitamin D is low, however, the levels of calcium and phosphorus in your blood drop and the body has no choice but to steal them from your bones. If this demineralization goes on long enough, osteomalacia, a disease in which bones become soft and misshapen, sets in. The disorder, also called "adult rickets," has a reputation for cruelty: It often brings bone pain, tenderness and muscle weakness.

But this loss of minerals can do more than soften bones: It can thin them as well, leaving them as brittle as dry sticks. A bump against a chair, a minor fall, even a coughing spell can crack such fragile bones. This malady's name is osteoporosis; its calling card is low back pain, loss of body height and fractures.

Take away vitamin D and the neuromuscular system can recoil with the signs of tetany: cramps, muscle twitching, convulsions and spasms of the wrist and ankle joints. A fibrillating (twitching) heart is another possible sign of a D deficiency.

ARE YOU LOW ON D?

But how likely is it that your body's D reserves will run low? Many people assume that everyone gets more than enough D from sunshine or fortified milk. But the reports of D deficiency keep coming in.

One is from the University of New Mexico School of Medicine in Albuquerque. John L. Omdahl, Ph.D., and his colleagues conducted a five-year study there to evaluate levels of vitamin D in nearly 300 older men and women. To find out how much D the subjects were getting, the researchers analyzed their diets and checked their blood levels of the major circulating form of vitamin D, 25-hydroxyvitamin D, or 25-OHD for short.

At the beginning of the study the researchers figured that if any group of older people had adequate levels of D, this one did. After all, they had decent incomes, were free of major illness and maintained a keen interest in their health. But when the data came in, it brought a surprise with it.

Most of the group had 25-OHD levels that were relatively low, and *over half* the group showed vitamin D intakes lower than 200 I.U., the Recommended Dietary Allowance for their age. In fact, one-third of them got less than 100 I.U. per day.

"This was a healthy population we were looking at," Dr. Omdahl says. "Yet their vitamin D status was poor, especially among the women. We think that deficiencies in elderly people who aren't as lucky as our subjects—those in institutions or those who don't get much sun—are probably even more prevalent. At any rate, it seems that the dietary intakes of the elderly in the United States may be somewhat lower than the RDA."

THE AGING FACTOR

There may be more to their vitamin D deficiency than lack of ultraviolet light and low D intake, say some researchers. The metabolic minuet of vitamin D may actually falter with age: Intestinal absorption of D may get out of adjustment, and the liver may not handle the nutrient as well as it should.

In addition, older people suffer a slowdown in the skin's D synthesis, according to Michael F. Holick, M.D., Ph.D., of the department of medicine at Harvard Medical School. "It's pretty clear," Dr. Holick says, "that after age 40 or 50 there is a steady decline in the skin's ability to produce previtamin D_3, the precursor of vitamin D. The skin of a 70-year-old can make about half the vitamin D_3 precursor produced by a 20-year-old.

Vitamin D-Rich Recipe: Salmon Cucumber Soup

Makes 4 to 6 servings

8 ounces cooked salmon
4 small cucumbers
1 cup chicken, vegetable or fish broth
1 medium onion, chopped
2 tablespoons lemon juice

2 teaspoons minced dill or ½ teaspoon dried dill
1 cup plain yogurt
toasted sesame seeds (garnish)
paprika (garnish)

Flake the salmon. Peel cucumbers if they have been waxed and cut them into chunks. Place salmon with broth, cucumbers and onion in blender or food processor. Blend until smooth. Add lemon juice and dill. Puree thoroughly. Stir in yogurt. Chill.

Serve in chilled bowls, garnished with toasted sesame seeds and paprika.

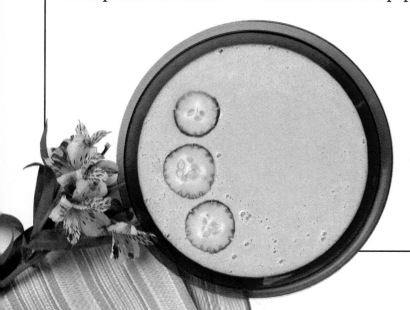

"We think, though, that the elderly may be able to compensate for this lowered production by getting more sunshine or vitamin D supplementation."

How much more? Experts agree that most healthy adults need at least 200 I.U. of D per day—from sun, supplements or food. For the elderly, though, vitamin D requirements may be higher. On the basis of their study, Dr. Omdahl and his colleagues suggest that in winter senior citizens should supplement their diets with about 400 I.U. a day—cod-liver oil or other D-rich fish-liver oils would be logical sources. And older people who don't get out in the summer sun should keep up that intake year-round. Elderly women, the researchers say, may need even higher intakes.

But the sky is definitely *not* the limit. Studies suggest that vitamin D in larger quantities can be highly toxic or ineffectual or both.

WINTER GIVES VITAMIN D THE COLD SHOULDER

But why can't people get their quota of D from old Sol? Actually, most people can. It's just that things sometimes get in the way of the D-making process.

Like winter, for instance. Bundling up for jaunts out in the cold north wind might keep you snug, but it won't help your skin catch a lot of rays. And sitting in a sunny window won't help your D reserves at all. Ultraviolet light can't penetrate ordinary window glass. And even if you sunbathed in the snow like an arctic seal, Old Man Winter would have you at a disadvantage. The low angle of the winter sun cuts out a lot of UVL.

"Under normal circumstances just 15 to 20 minutes of summer sun exposure per day would fulfill the vitamin D requirement of a lightly pigmented person," says Dr. Holick. "But that much exposure would be inadequate in the winter. The low-lying sun slants its rays through the ozone layer in the stratosphere, forcing the light to pass through more of that layer. The result is less

The Best Food Sources of Vitamin D

Food	Portion	Vitamin D (I.U.)
Halibut-liver oil	2 tsp.	11,200
Herring	3 oz.	840
Cod-liver oil	2 tsp.	800
Mackerel	3 oz.	708
Salmon, Pacific	3 oz.	420
Tuna	2 oz.	168

UVL reaching the earth."

Then you have that other sun filter to worry about—air pollution. Researchers think that in the years from 1951 to 1972, increased pollution cut our total vitamin D accumulation by 15 percent, and today we may receive even less.

If you have dark skin, you have a built-in sunscreen that can reduce your share of UVL. Heavily pigmented skin can stop as much as 95 percent of UVL from reaching the deep dermal layers where D is made. It's no wonder then that dark-skinned people in northern climes have more cases of rickets than their light-skinned neighbors.

But researchers have found that people who spend a fair amount of time outdoors during the summer actually build up a "pool" of vitamin D that *can* last through the winter. That's because vitamin D is fat soluble and is stored in the body. According to one study, schoolchildren who spent their summer vacations basking at the seashore had more vitamin D in their blood the following winter than did kids who spent the summer in town.

"There is evidence that even in winter, the concentration of circulating [vitamin D] in normal people is determined largely by exposure to solar radiation the previous summer," according to the *British Medical Journal*.

What this means to bone health was demonstrated in a study conducted in Leeds, England. Doctors

The big, yellow hump on this graph represents levels of sunlight through the year. The other curve shows levels of vitamin D in the body, which peak and dip in response to sun levels but lag slightly behind because the body takes a while to store or lose the nutrient. That's why the biggest plunge in D levels is in early spring, and why you might want to take a vitamin D supplement to protect your bones.

examined samples from the hipbones of 134 patients who had suffered suspicious fractures of the hipbone or thighbone over a period of five years. They concluded that 37 percent of the patients were suffering from osteomalacia. But what was most disturbing was the fact that by far the largest number of fractures occurred in the period from February through June.

"As would be expected if this seasonal variation was attributable to variation in the supply of vitamin D dependent on sunlight, the proportion of cases with osteomalacia is highest in the spring and lowest in the autumn," they noted.

So summer sun can be a friend. Excessive sunbathing, though, is unhealthy: It can wrinkle your skin prematurely and cause skin cancer. But moderate sunbathing may *prevent* cancer.

CAN SUNSHINE BEAT COLON CANCER?

Two scientists who conducted research at Johns Hopkins University in Baltimore have theorized that sunshine and a year-round supply of vitamin D might prevent colon cancer.

"We have simply shown," says one of the researchers, Cedric F. Garland, Ph.D., "that there is a predilection for colon cancer in areas that receive less sunlight."

Dr. Garland and his brother, Frank Garland, Ph.D., made that discovery while comparing the rates of colon cancer and skin cancer in the United States. In the Sun Belt, skin cancer was common but colon cancer wasn't. In the colder regions, the reverse was true. Intrigued, they borrowed sunshine statistics from

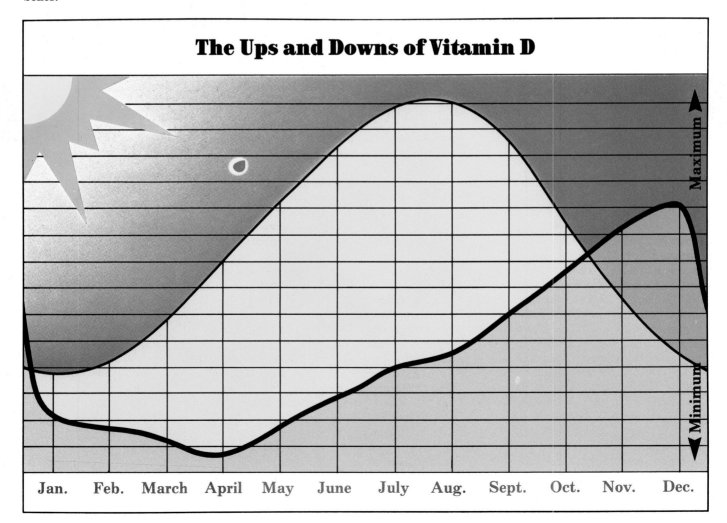

The Ups and Downs of Vitamin D

| Jan. | Feb. | March | April | May | June | July | Aug. | Sept. | Oct. | Nov. | Dec. |

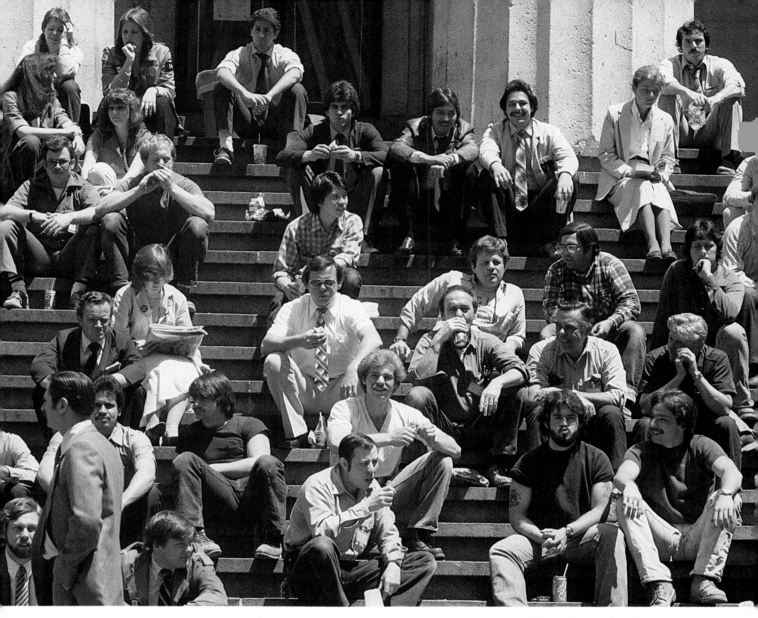

the U.S. Weather Service. The numbers pointed to an inverse relationship between sunshine and colon cancer. A cattleman in sunny, sparsely populated New Mexico, for example, is much less likely to get colon cancer than a stockbroker in smoggy, crowded New York. Per 100,000 people, 17.3 New Yorkers will suffer from colon cancer, but only 6.7 New Mexicans will.

Inhabitants of cities are deprived of sunshine for several reasons. Ozone pollution deflects some of the urban sunlight. Tall buildings eclipse the sun even more. "Even in areas where sunlight is intense," Dr. Cedric Garland has written, "persons who live and work in cities may not receive much exposure to it. . . . Vitamin D deficiency occurs in large cities even in tropical and sub-

tropical areas."

How do the researchers think vitamin D protects the colon? Working with the known fact that vitamin D enables the body to absorb calcium, they theorize that calcium's presence somehow protects the lining of the colon from cancer-causing waste substances that pass through it.

In the future, the doctors plan to survey vitamin D levels in Americans, asking such questions as: Do lifeguards have more vitamin D than lawyers? How much does outdoor recreation contribute to the vitamin D supply?

So, while no one is suggesting you overdo the tanning, it might be a good idea to at least get outside regularly when the sun beckons.

Even the people who aren't eating lunch or snacking are "eating" vitamin D by sitting outside, because this vitamin is formed when the sun's ultraviolet rays hit the skin. But these sunbathing New Yorkers may still need a supplement to get their daily quota of the nutrient: "If you live in a smoggy city or in the shadows of tall buildings, you may have just as much trouble getting enough vitamin D as someone who stays indoors all the time," says Frank Konishi, Ph.D., coordinator of dietetics at Southern Illinois University.

7

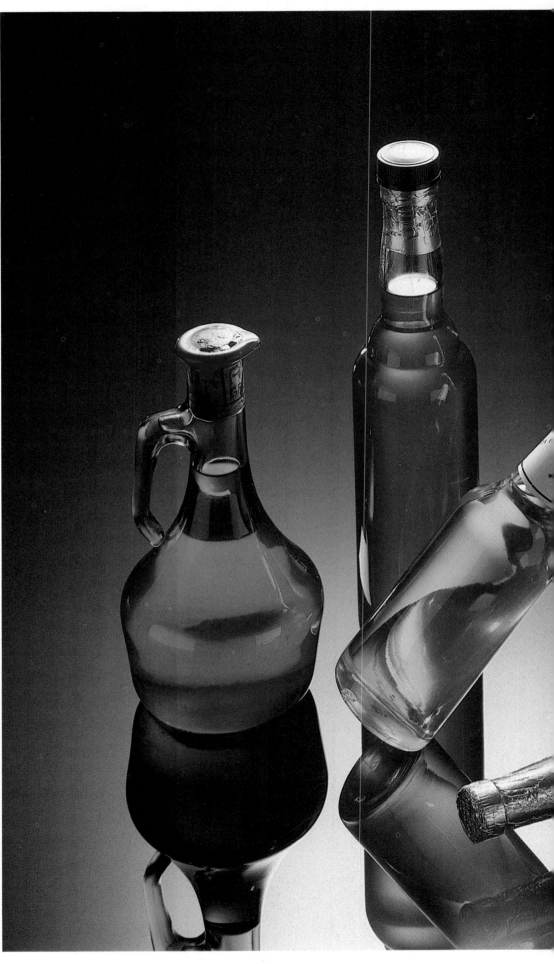

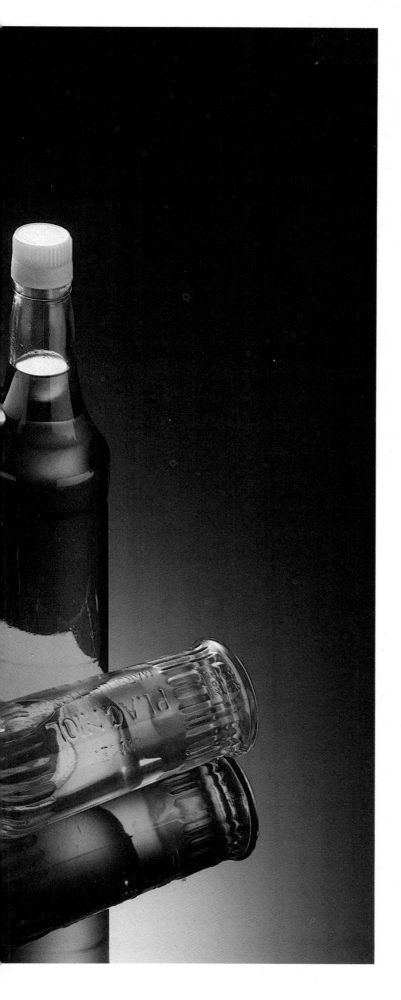

Vitamin E: Strong Medicine

Once the "vitamin in search of a deficiency," it's now lauded as a force that slows aging and strengthens the heart.

Scientists are finding that vitamin E is a nutritional Swiss Army knife. The Swiss have a knack for making the greatest use of the smallest space, and with one of their military's pocketknives you can open cans, uncork bottles, clip your nails, practically everything short of balancing your checkbook and squaring the circle.

While the knife's amazing, it's nothing next to vitamin E. Everyone knows what vitamin E can do for your circulation: It modifies blood fats so that they protect against heart disease. Vitamin E also may promote a healthy circulatory system by preventing the formation of dangerous blood clots and by protecting red blood cells from damage by oxidation.

If vitamin E worked just to prevent heart disease, it would be impressive enough. But on top of that, scientists are finding that this vitamin protects health in other ways as well.

In fact, at a meeting in New York City held by the New York Academy of Sciences, vitamin E experts from all over the world gathered for three days to swap notes they'd been jotting down for ten years or more.

Armed with speeches, slides, graphs and charts, they all testified to the fact that vitamin E is no longer a "vitamin in search of a deficiency," as it had been called. Instead, it's a vitamin that can influence many illnesses and provides a key to the healthy functioning of our muscles, eyes, blood, lungs and more.

The variety of E's protective action is most astonishing. It boosts our immune system so that we are better protected from viruses, bacterial diseases and, in some cases, cancer. It even keeps the sparkle in our eyes. For example, it has been shown that animals given large doses of vitamin E don't develop certain kinds of cataracts. It's been shown, too, that vitamin E may enhance our resistance to an ever-worsening threat to health: pollution. How can one substance do *all* those things?

Vitamin E-Rich Recipe: Pumpkin Muffins

Makes 2 dozen

1 cup honey
½ cup oil
4 eggs
1½ cups cooked pumpkin
2¾ cups whole wheat
    flour, sifted
¼ cup wheat germ
1½ teaspoons baking
    powder
1 teaspoon baking soda

½ teaspoon ground
    cloves
¾ teaspoon ground
    cinnamon
½ teaspoon ground
    nutmeg
1½ cups raisins
1 cup walnuts, coarsely
    chopped

Place honey, oil, eggs and pumpkin in a bowl and mix. Sift together flour, wheat germ, baking powder, baking soda and spices. Add dry ingredients to wet ingredients and mix. Add raisins and walnuts. Divide batter evenly in greased muffin tins and bake at 400°F for 15 minutes. Let cool 5 minutes and remove from tins.

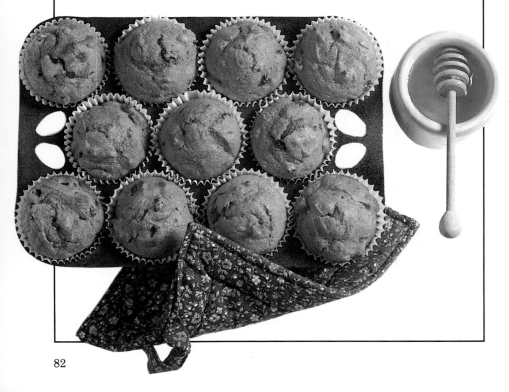

HOW VITAMIN E HELPS THE BODY

To understand what vitamin E does you need to know a little bit about oxygen. Obviously, you can't live without it. But each breath you take, drenching every cell in your body with life-sustaining oxygen, carries you one step closer to old age. You see, the fats present in all cells can combine with oxygen at an excessive rate in a chemical process known as oxidation.

Given favorable conditions, oxidation will turn a shiny metal wrench into an ugly, rusted wrench very quickly. Our bodies, of course, don't rust. But under the right circumstances, oxidative damage produces the kind of accelerated wear and tear that may lead to premature aging, lowered resistance, cancer and heart disease.

Fortunately, nature has provided us with a way of slowing down such reactions. Cells and tissues are protected against oxidation in a variety of ways, but perhaps the most important are substances called antioxidants, which prevent, or at least slow down, the process of oxidation. These antioxidants exist in our bodies, so as long as the supply of antioxidants lasts, these damaging reactions are instantly checked. But one antioxidant molecule can stop only one damaging reaction. That means that a constant, "self-regenerating" supply is needed.

Luckily, one of the most important natural antioxidants is readily available. It's vitamin E.

To understand how vitamin E and other antioxidants protect us, let's take a look at some scientific findings.

On the most basic level, it appears that antioxidants can extend the life of cells. When clusters of rat brain cells are cultured in a test tube, they normally show signs of severe structural degeneration within 40 days. But when similar cell clusters were held in a culture supplemented with vitamin E, the cells were still well preserved and structurally sound after 40 days.

"The difference was like night and day," Bruce D. Trapp, Ph.D., of the National Institute of Neurological and Communicative Disorders and Stroke, says. According to Dr. Trapp, the cells lived longer because vitamin E may help preserve the cell membrane, letting various healthful substances into cells while letting wastes escape.

Besides slowing the aging process, antioxidants can block the formation of tumors. Thirty-three weeks after exposure to a powerful cancer-causing chemical, animals whose diets were supplemented with a mixture of four antioxidants— including vitamin E—developed only about half as many tumors as unprotected animals.

Antioxidants also appear to play a key role in fostering immunity, the body's natural ability to repel invading disease organisms. According to Werner A. Baumgartner, Ph.D., and co-workers in the nuclear medicine department at the Wadsworth Veterans' Administration Hospital in Los Angeles, body stores of vitamin E tend to fall sharply when there is a tumor. And this antioxidant deficiency may be responsible in part for the depressed immunity so common in cancer patients. The researchers suggest that adding extra antioxidants to the diets of cancer patients might reverse this often fatal situation.

"In fact," Dr. Baumgartner says, "there is growing evidence that even in healthy people the immune processes require more antioxidants than we normally take in with our food. The immune system seems to require *more* antioxidants than other cells in the body. So even a slight stress, such as a marginal deficiency of vitamin E, could impair the immune response."

In still another area, dermatologists report that they have found vitamin E to be of great therapeutic value in many disabling and stubborn skin disorders. And they believe the reason is vitamin E's antioxidant properties.

You even find vitamin E doing its miracles in your blood vessels and in your eyes. For instance, vitamin E may be the first line of defense against an eye problem called dia-

The Best Food Sources of Vitamin E

Food	Portion	Vitamin E (I.U.)
Wheat germ oil	1 tbsp.	37.2
Sunflower seeds	¼ cup	26.8
Wheat germ, raw	½ cup	12.8
Sunflower seed oil	1 tbsp.	12.7
Almonds	¼ cup	12.7
Pecans, halves	¼ cup	12.5
Hazelnuts	¼ cup	12.0
Safflower oil	1 tbsp.	7.9
Peanuts	¼ cup	4.9
Corn oil	1 tbsp.	4.8
Cod-liver oil	1 tbsp.	3.9
Peanut butter	2 tbsp.	3.8
Corn oil margarine	1 tbsp.	3.6
Soybean oil	1 tbsp.	3.5
Peanut oil	1 tbsp.	3.4
Lobster	3 oz.	2.3
Salmon steak	3 oz.	2.0

betic retinopathy, in which blood vessels in the eyes break, sometimes causing blindness.

More specifically, W. Gerald Robinson Jr., Ph.D., chief of the experimental anatomy section, laboratory of vision research, National Eye Institute, has been examining the effects on animal retinas of diets deficient in vitamins E and A. Results? "A highly E-deficient animal will go blind in time," he says.

To gain all those benefits from vitamin E, you must be certain that your diet provides adequate amounts. What is adequate? The Recommended Dietary Allowance according to the government's National Research Council is 12 I.U. for women and 15 I.U. for men, but research seems to show that the RDA—what is normally considered "enough" vitamin E—is far too low.

According to Cheryl Nockels, Ph.D., a Colorado State University scientist working with laboratory animals to determine the relationship between vitamin E and the immune function, "The RDA does not appear to maintain immunity at full strength. In every case, I found that an amount of vitamin E greater

In the blood, cholesterol is transported by complexes of fats and proteins called lipoproteins. Low-density lipoproteins (LDL) are "bad guys"—they carry cholesterol *to* the cells. High-density lipoproteins (HDL) are "good guys"—they carry cholesterol *away* from the cells. A high percentage of LDL in the total cholesterol means a high risk of circulatory disease like heart attack or stroke. A high percentage of HDL means a low risk. In this study, William Hermann, M.D., a pathologist at Memorial City General Hospital in Houston, gave 600 to 800 I.U. of vitamin E per day to 5 people with very low HDL. After a month or more of taking the nutrient, their cholesterol was normal—and their chance of a heart attack or stroke much less.

than the RDA for the [experimental] animal was required to stimulate improved immune response," she says.

The daily amounts of vitamin E recommended by researchers vary anywhere from 100 to 600 I.U. But there are probably no harmful effects from taking 800 I.U. a day for many years, a study has shown, so you can use vitamin E with confidence.

Of course, even if you take a supplement, you still want to get as much vitamin E from your food as you're entitled to. And it's simple to do: Avoid overprocessed and refined foods.

Canned and frozen foods lose up to 65 percent of their vitamin E. Grains are a good source, at least until they're milled. Cornflakes, for instance, have lost 98 percent of their vitamin E. Whole grain wheat has more than ten times the vitamin E in bleached white flour and brown rice

has more than five times the amount in white rice. Nuts, another good source, may lose about 28 percent of their vitamin E when dry-roasted. Oils, too, provide plenty of vitamin E, especially wheat germ oil and sunflower seed oil. To get the most vitamin E, eat whole foods.

CLEAR VEINS, STRONG HEART

It's probably safe to say that most of us don't give much thought to our circulatory system when we're feeling great. We just take it for granted that our blood will flow through our veins as smoothly as water through pipes.

But sometimes things don't work out as problem free as planned. Telltale symptoms may begin to crop up, signaling trouble. With pipes it's pretty easy to see when something is wrong. If the water drains slowly, there's probably debris building up inside. Time to break out the Drāno or call Roto-Rooter.

But what if your *arteries* or *veins* are clogging up?

Narrowed blood vessels can lead to high blood pressure, angina, heart attack, thrombophlebitis (inflammation of a vein associated with a blood clot) or even circulatory ulcers of the feet. And there's no plumber to fix this disaster. Instead, it's best to keep your blood vessels from narrowing in the first place. That's where vitamin E comes in.

As we mentioned earlier, blood usually flows through our veins without difficulty. But sometimes the vessel walls can narrow, either because of fat buildup (atherosclerosis) or from blood platelets clumping up at the wrong time against the inside of the vessel wall. (Platelets are tiny disk-shaped elements essential for clotting, or stopping the flow of blood, in the event of a cut. They can *over*clot, however, increasing the risk of heart disease.) For both of those sticky problems, vitamin E can be a lifesaver.

The problem of atherosclerosis stems directly from cholesterol in our diet. You probably are aware that high cholesterol levels in the blood constitute an important risk factor: They can lead to atherosclerotic

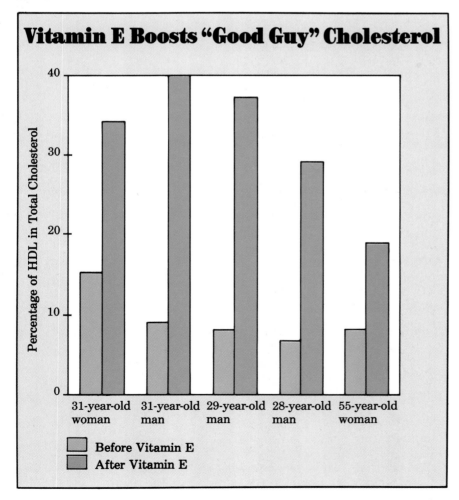

Vitamin E Boosts "Good Guy" Cholesterol

Percentage of HDL in Total Cholesterol

- 31-year-old woman
- 31-year-old man
- 29-year-old man
- 28-year-old man
- 55-year-old woman

Before Vitamin E
After Vitamin E

damage to blood vessel walls that may further lead to heart attack or stroke. But not inevitably. When cholesterol is hooked up with high-density lipoproteins (HDL), it's relatively harmless. But combine it with low-density lipoproteins (LDL), and you've got a problem: Cholesterol's on a rampage. That's why scientists now think that taking care of total cholesterol is less important than keeping HDL levels as high as possible. And that is just what vitamin E does.

This point was demonstrated in an experiment conducted by William J. Hermann, Jr., M.D., a pathologist at Memorial City General Hospital in Houston. He picked five people with average amounts of HDL cholesterol and five with low HDL levels and placed them all on 600 I.U. of vitamin E per day. Within a few weeks, all five people with cholesterol problems increased their HDL levels between 220 and 483 percent. Even four of the five people with average levels saw their HDL fractions rise as much as 237 percent.

The effect of the vitamin E appears to be a redistribution of cholesterol, say Dr. Hermann and his colleagues, that elevates the HDL fraction and decreases the LDL part.

The magnitude of the change in the high-risk group may possibly indicate a deficiency of vitamin E that originally contributed to their abnormal levels of HDL and LDL cholesterol, according to the researchers.

That kind of discovery is very important to people who, for some reason, aren't able to lace themselves into jogging shoes, slip into low-coefficient-of-drag running shorts and beat the pavement for 10 or more miles every week. As many people know, exercise causes HDL cholesterol levels to go up. But not everyone can jog. For those people, vitamin E provides an effective alternative.

In fact, vitamin E works best for those who need it most. People who have the lowest levels of HDL tend to experience the most dramatic improvement when they take vitamin E.

Such was the finding in experiments at the Wood Veterans' Admin-istration Hospital in Milwaukee, where a team of researchers supplemented 43 volunteers, ranging in age from 22 to 60, with 800 I.U. of vitamin E per day for four weeks.

Of the 43, 30 were men and 13 were women. Seventeen of the men, suffering from spinal cord injuries, had unusually low HDL levels. Of the 13 healthy men, 8 jogged regularly or ran long-distance races, and they enjoyed relatively high HDL levels. After one month of supplementation, the women, the nonjogging men and the men with spinal cord injuries who initially had very low HDL levels improved the most.

"There's no question that vitamin E is important in a number of ways," one of the researchers reported. "But as far as cholesterol goes, we were looking for even more reliable proof. With the small study we've done with 43 people, not one

Calf cramps while walking— also called intermittent claudication—are often caused by poor circulation in the lower leg. In this study, people with cramping were divided into 2 groups: one took vitamin E and the other (the control group) didn't. The E group had a big improvement in circulation, while the control group got a little worse.

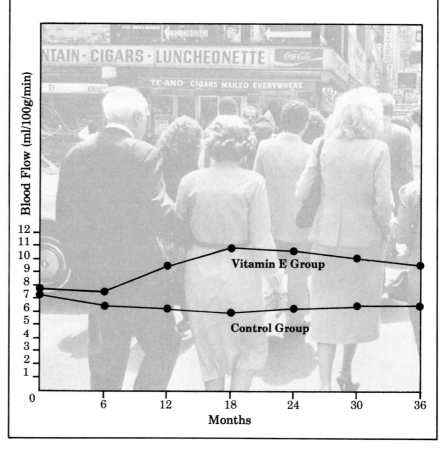

Calf Cramps while Walking? Vitamin E Takes Them in Stride

Vitamin E Group

Control Group

Blood Flow (ml/100g/min)

Months

noticed any negative side effects. On the contrary, one of the women said that her dry skin condition cleared up while she was taking the vitamin.

"We know that exercise can raise HDL levels, but not everyone, and certainly not every heart patient, is able to exercise," the researchers said.

In addition to balancing the HDL and LDL in our arteries' favor, vitamin E fights the fat in another way.

Researchers from the department of internal medicine at Kyoto University in Japan conducted a study to examine the effect of vitamin E on lipid peroxidation. (Lipid peroxides

are fat oxidation products that are toxic to human and animal tissues. It's suspected that when they accumulate in blood vessels they impair circulation by promoting atherosclerosis and blood clots.)

The researchers found that animals fed a diet deficient in vitamin E actually produced significantly *more* of these peroxides than did a group supplemented with vitamin E.

The good news here is that the damage created by the vitamin E deficiency was reversible. The results support the possibility, cited by the researchers, that administration of vitamin E could prevent or lessen damage to the blood vessels, even some of the vandalism caused by an accumulation of lipid peroxides.

J. C. Alexander, Ph.D., would heartily agree. He's done his own experiments, at the University of Guelph in Ontario, on the effects of vitamin E on oxidized fats.

"Accumulation of oxidized fats in tissues can have a toxic effect," Dr. Alexander says. "It certainly did with our experimental animals. We saw evidence of cellular damage to kidney, heart and liver tissues.

"In this particular experiment, we used cells taken from the hearts of laboratory animals to test the influence of vitamins E and C on the biological effects of oxidized fats. These vitamins (probably in their role as antioxidants) counteracted the adverse effects, such as excessive lipid accumulation, in the heart cells.

"This is especially important," explains Dr. Alexander, "because there is evidence that oxidized lipids can accelerate symptoms of vitamin E deficiency.

"People who eat a lot of fried foods are particularly vulnerable, because frying allows oxidation of fats to take place faster," Dr. Alexander says. "What's more, a diet like that may be deficient in vitamin E, compounding the problem. That's especially true of teenagers, who are known to eat a lot of fried or fatty foods—like hamburgers, hot dogs and fries.

"There is no doubt in my mind that vitamin E is a potent antioxidant and extremely important in maintaining a healthy circulatory system," he says. "Anyone who

What Is Platelet Aggregation?

Platelets are tiny cells that normally slip freely through the blood (the photo at right shows normal platelets). If they grow sticky and clump together, or aggregate (like those in the photo below), the result may be a dangerous clot in a blood vessel. Fortunately, vitamin E decreases platelet aggregation.

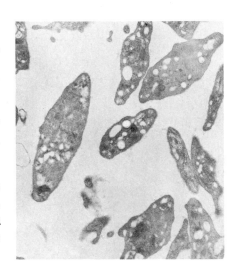

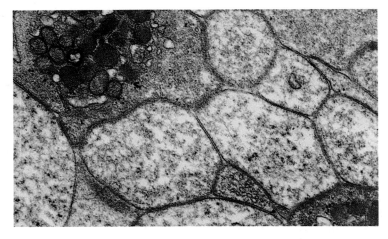

doesn't believe that is fooling himself."

Believer or not, we'll tell you how vitamin E has also been shown to lower the risk of buildup on arterial walls by keeping your platelets from clumping up.

DISSOLVING BLOOD CLOTS

When hospital patients are fed intravenously, they are particularly susceptible to vitamin E deficiency and the problems that go with it, such as excessively sticky platelets.

According to Peter M. Thurlow, M.D., and John P. Grant, M.D., of the department of surgery at Duke University Medical Center in Durham, North Carolina, a deficiency can be a real threat in such cases. They studied 13 patients whose total nourishment was given intravenously for two weeks or more. This type of feeding, along with standard vitamin supplementation, is associated with a gradual decrease in the amount of vitamin E in the blood, say Dr. Thurlow and Dr. Grant.

And as serum vitamin E levels decrease, platelet aggregation (a scientific phrase for clotting) becomes abnormal. One patient whose vitamin E concentration and platelet aggregation were initially normal developed a deficiency and platelet hyperaggregation (overly sticky platelets) after 15 days of intravenous feeding.

In fact, every patient with a low vitamin E level also had abnormal platelet aggregation. Supplementation raised the plasma vitamin E levels and returned platelet aggregation to normal in most of those patients.

While all of us should guard our blood vessels, people with diabetes need to show even greater concern. Not only does a diabetic's body fail to regulate the amount of sugar in the blood, but, as a group, diabetics run a higher than normal risk of developing heart disease. Vitamin E seems to work in two ways. It helps prevent abnormal clotting, and it also lowers the amount of sugar in the blood.

That's a conclusion reached by Marvin L. Bierenbaum, M.D., of the Atherosclerosis Research Group in Montclair, New Jersey. When Dr. Bierenbaum gave 2,000 I.U. of vitamin E per day for six weeks to a group of 25 diabetics, their blood sugar levels fell by 6 percent, a change significant enough to make him announce his finding at an American Heart Association convention. Dr. Bierenbaum also noted that those patients' blood platelets became slightly less inclined to stick together and form clots.

That anticlotting ability makes vitamin E a potentially lifesaving tool in surgery. All surgery carries with it the risk that a clot (called a thrombus or embolism) will form and block a blood vessel, thereby cutting off vital blood flow. If that happens, a heart attack or stroke can follow. According to a survey of surgeons in England, 2 percent of the elderly people who have a hip replacement die from a pulmonary embolism — that is, a clot that blocks blood flow to the lungs.

In spite of the risks of clot formation, many doctors either do not take precautions against it or else use prescription blood thinners that carry with them a list of side effects. But a few surgeons over the years have used vitamin E.

One of those pioneers was Alton Ochsner, M.D., of Tulane University in New Orleans. Dr. Ochsner has written that he routinely gave vitamin E to every patient he treated for a major injury of any kind, and rarely did any of them ever develop a pulmonary embolism. Dr. Ochsner prescribed from 200 to 600 I.U. of vitamin E per day, starting no later than the day of surgery and continuing well into the healing stage.

Actually, that's probably good advice for just about everyone, not just those recovering from surgery. Clear, open blood vessels mean healthier circulation, no matter what your present state of health.

SMOG, STRESS AND VITAMIN E

We're all swimming in a sea of stress. Physical, emotional, chemical. But some of us are in over our heads.

Air pollution is dragging our lungs down for the third time. Some scientists say that radiation—

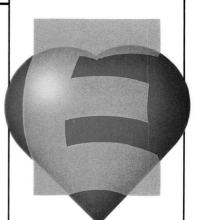

Easing Angina

Searing, stabbing pain. Angina. It's helped by drugs. But some research suggests high doses of vitamin E may help, too. T. W. Anderson, M.D., Ph.D., of the University of British Columbia, studied 15 angina patients who'd been taking vitamin E for some time. Without their knowledge, 7 people were given fake pills (with no vitamin E). In 3 weeks, 3 people had to quit the trial because their angina returned with a vengeance. People still taking E, though, had no such experience.

microwaves, X rays, nuclear power—is a hidden riptide of stress that can wash our health out to sea.

Do you have a sinking feeling about all that stress? Then swim—with vitamin E.

When researchers want to find out about stress, they don't kid around. One of their favorite tests is to put rats into a tub of cold water and see how long they can swim before sinking. The test packs a lifetime of stress into an hour (the rats even develop ulcers).

A researcher from the California State University in Hayward conducted such a test. But first he divided the rats into a few groups, and for 18 days supplemented the diet of some groups with vitamin E. He found that the vitamin E rats swam longer and had milder ulcers than the animals who weren't fed vitamin E.

But does this test hold water for you? After all, you're probably not a member of the local Polar Bear Club. But you are someone who breathes, and that means coping with a source of stress that can give cold feet to anyone who's striving for better health—air pollution. Vitamin E can guard against that, too.

Daniel Menzel, Ph.D., a researcher at the Duke University Medical Center, continuously exposed three groups of mice to ozone, one of the deadliest air pollutants. One group, however, received a large amount of vitamin E with its diet, another group got a smaller amount and the third group got no vitamin E. The group receiving the large amount of vitamin E survived an average of two weeks longer than the other groups.

In another experiment, Dr. Menzel exposed two groups of mice to nitrogen dioxide, a pollutant just as deadly as ozone. He gave one group a daily amount of vitamin E equivalent to what a person would get if he took a 100 I.U. supplement. The other group received the equivalent of 10 I.U. of vitamin E, the amount found in the average American's diet. After three months of exposure to nitrogen dioxide, both groups of mice had lung damage "very similar to what occurs in the early stages of human emphysema,"

says Dr. Menzel. But the 100 I.U. mice had significantly less lung damage.

Well, you're not a mouse. But you are a guinea pig in an experiment called the 20th century—continuous exposure to ozone, nitrogen dioxide and a menacing mix of other air pollutants. And you don't want to be in the 10 I.U. group—even if you live where the air *seems* clean.

"Air pollution is not confined to metropolitan areas," Dr. Menzel says. "The amount of ozone in certain rural areas of New Jersey is greater than in downtown Manhattan."

To protect his own health, Dr. Menzel takes 200 I.U. of vitamin E every day.

In another study on ozone and vitamin E, Mohammad G. Mustafa, Ph.D., associate professor of public health and medicine at the University of California at Los Angeles, divided rats into two groups, feeding one group a diet containing 11 parts per million (ppm) of vitamin E and the other group a diet with 66 ppm. After five weeks on these diets, the animals were exposed to ozone for a week.

After the ozone exposure, the researcher inspected the animals' lungs. The rats receiving the smaller amounts of vitamin E had more lung damage than the better-supplemented rats.

The rats on the low vitamin E diet received about the same concentration of the vitamin found in the average American diet, Dr. Mustafa points out. That level was *not* enough to protect the animals' lungs. "The findings may be of relevance to human population exposed to photochemical smog," he concludes.

Too little vitamin E in our diet may make us vulnerable to air pollution in more ways than one, other evidence suggests. Besides damaging the lungs, ozone can also harm red blood cells, which carry life-sustaining oxygen to the tissues of the body.

When researchers at the University of Kentucky and the University of California at Davis fed rats a diet deficient in vitamin E and then exposed them to atmospheric concentrations of 0.8 ppm of ozone, red cells showed significant damage. But cells of other animals fed supplemental vitamin E emerged unscathed.

"During continuous exposure to or contact with various types of noxious agents in the cellular environment," the investigators note, "the metabolic machinery of the red cells is able to reverse most of the adverse effects of the insult under normal conditions." However, "when the defense capability is reduced, as might occur in nutritional inadequacy, significant or irreversible changes in the red cells may result." Fortunately, they conclude, vitamin E appears to occupy "a unique place" in bolstering that defense.

Why can't your body go it alone against air pollution? Oxidation is why. As discussed earlier, oxidation slowly scorches our cells. Add ozone and nitrogen dioxide, and the scorch of oxidation can turn into a four-alarm blaze. Fortunately, vitamin E douses the fire.

But that's not the whole story.

Free radicals are chemical maniacs, out-of-control molecules that roam around looking for something to destroy. Oxidation creates the free radicals and they do the dirty work—but not if they meet their match in vitamin E. Oxidation isn't the only process that creates free radicals, however. So does radiation.

Radiation—the energy that beams out of X ray machines and pulses at the core of nuclear reactors. Like an atom-sized bullet racing at nearly the speed of light, radiation can rip into the very center of a cell. The wound is called cancer. Some scientists believe that free radicals play a major role in this shoot-out. And with various kinds of radiation in the living room (color TV), the bedroom (luminous clock dial) and the kitchen (microwave oven), vitamin E may help keep your home a sweet home.

Researchers from the Netherlands grew cell cultures in their laboratory, adding vitamin E to some of the cultures. After several weeks, they bombarded all the cells with X rays—and more of the cells cultured with vitamin E survived.

Radiation is a typically modern—and typically dangerous—stress, but vitamin E takes it on. And it even tussles with the toughest customer there is—aging.

TEN MORE YEARS OF LIFE

In a study on vitamin E and aging, Jeffrey Bland, Ph.D., a scientist from Tacoma, Washington, took blood samples from 24 men and women and exposed the blood cells to oxidation. Almost all of the cells were severely damaged. He then gave each of the 24 people 600 I.U. of vitamin E a day, and after ten days again took blood samples and exposed the cells to oxidation. The second time, almost all of the cells remained completely intact.

"Greater amounts of vitamin E in the diet can help to prevent the cells of our bodies from aging faster than necessary," Dr. Bland says. He recommends between 100 and 400 I.U. of vitamin E a day, not only to help keep cells young, but also to protect the whole body from smog, radiation and other types of stress.

A scientist who agrees with Dr. Bland is Denham Harman, M.D., Ph.D., a professor at the University of Nebraska College of Medicine in Omaha and the chief proponent of the theory that free radicals are to blame for aging. (He also says that cancer, heart disease, high blood pressure and senility are all caused, in part, by free radicals.) According to Dr. Harman, a diet that includes ample amounts of vitamin E could "lessen the possibility of those health problems occurring." Such a diet, he adds, "may reasonably be expected to add five to ten or more years of healthy, productive life to the life span of the average person."

VITAMIN E AND WOUND HEALING

Now we're going to tell you how vitamin E has enhanced the chances for healthy survival for the members of one of the fastest-growing clubs in America—the Ostomates. Membership in this club is restricted to those who have undergone surgery involving substitute routes for elimination of body wastes. We're going to tell you about a team of surgeons and a

Mercury

Yearly, 310 tons of toxic mercury pollute our air; 80 tons go into our water. But vitamin E may help: In a study by toxicologists, animals exposed to mercury had severe brain and nerve damage. But animals that got mercury plus vitamin E ended up in almost perfect health.

310 Tons

80 Tons

nurse therapist who, working together in a spirit of cooperation, have been able to make the Pottsville Hospital in Pennsylvania just about the best place to go if you are anticipating this kind of surgery.

John L. Flanigan, Jr., M.D., a surgeon, is director of the hospital's enterostomal therapy department. Dorothy Fisher was the head enterostomal therapist. (She is now retired.)

Enterostomal therapy is a specialty that developed out of the very special need of the patient who undergoes the kind of surgery that necessitates an opening (stoma) in the abdomen. Colostomy is one procedure, ileostomy and urinary diversion are others. The opening in the body is very susceptible to infection and often resistant to healing, and it sometimes causes more trouble than the surgery or condition that necessitated it. That's why nurses like Mrs. Fisher are trained in enterostomal therapy so they can better the cure rate after this kind of surgery.

Dismayed by the pain, agony and slow healing often encountered in stomal patients and ulceration cases, Mrs. Fisher was highly motivated in her search for a solution to the problems. She devoured all the literature on the subject of skin healing, and was excited by reports

about quick healing of this distressing type of wound when vitamin E is used.

"We believe that Pottsville Hospital uses more vitamin E by mouth than any hospital in the state and maybe any in the country," she says. "There are several physicians on the staff of the Pottsville Hospital prescribing vitamin E. They don't waste time using small amounts anymore. Twelve hundred I.U. is the minimum we start with. Some surgeons order 400 I.U. to be given four times a day. And they get marvelous results!

"In one case, a badly ulcerated stoma was completely healed in seven days—which is phenomenal considering the deficiencies of the patient, who was in a very poor state of nutrition."

Three days after this patient's surgery, which was performed for rectal cancer with a resultant sigmoid colostomy stoma, the area of the stoma was ulcerating. The surgeon was dismayed and considered reopening the wound.

"Why don't we see first what we can do with vitamin E," Mrs. Fisher urged. "Give us three days." Then she set to work. She treated the stoma and the area around it every day with vitamin E oil (60 I.U. per gram). "We practically drowned it in vitamin E oil. And we gave the patient 400 I.U. of natural vitamin E orally four times a day. The patient made a fantastic recovery in a week and no further surgery was necessary."

SMOOTH, NO-PROBLEM SKIN

Vitamin E isn't only for healing. It also does good things for the way you look.

Leo Roy, M.D., of Toronto, thinks that a person with dry skin might benefit from fresh wheat germ oil, which supplies not only oil but also vitamin E.

Max Vogel, M.D., of Calgary, Alberta, gives patients with dry skin vitamin E: "Four hundred I.U. two times a day—with breakfast and supper," he says.

In fact, most of the doctors we talked to about dry, red, rough skin (and most of the doctors we talked to

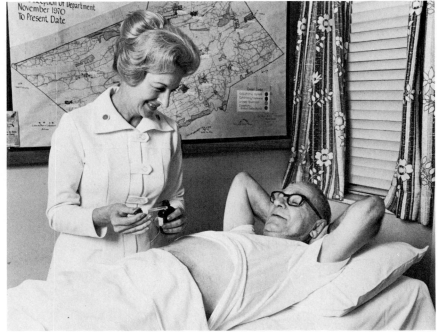

While a nurse therapist at Pottsville Hospital in Pennsylvania, Dorothy Fisher (now retired) applied vitamin E oil to the surgical wounds of many patients. Doctors at the hospital also prescribe the vitamin, which Mrs. Fisher says speeds healing and has even cleared up serious ulcerations that would have required additional surgery.

were from Canada, where the winters really skin you alive) also recommended using vitamin oils *on* the skin.

"I have my patients with dry skin take vitamin E oil by mouth and also put it on the dry area," says Gerald Green, M.D., of Toronto.

"My patients use a mixture of vitamin E and vitamins A and D ointment on cracked lips and dry skin," says Dr. Vogel.

But vitamin E is strong medicine. Strong enough to tackle more than just dry skin.

Consider discoid lupus erythematosus (DLE), for example. It's a chronic disease of the skin that torments its victims with red, circular blotches or plaques. Pore openings widen and become plugged with scale. DLE can be quite an ordeal.

That's why a report by two Los Angeles dermatologists, Samuel Ayres Jr., M.D., and Richard Mihan, M.D., is so noteworthy. Dr. Ayres, a former clinical professor of medicine at UCLA, and Dr. Mihan, of the University of Southern California School of Medicine, have had excellent results treating DLE patients with vitamin E. "It must be employed in a potent form, in adequate amounts, and over an extended period of time, sometimes indefinitely, to achieve maximum therapeutic benefits," they say.

Dr. Ayres and Dr. Mihan describe two patients treated with vitamin E. One, a 63-year-old woman, had been troubled by discoid lupus for about eight months. Reddish, scaly and crusty blotches the size of nickels and quarters marred her skin. She was given high doses of vitamin E daily, and a special cream containing vitamin E was applied directly to the skin twice a day. "Five and a half months later, the patient's skin was completely cleared," the doctors report. "Her response was excellent."

Another woman, 37 years old, had suffered with lupus symptoms on and off for 23 years. Pea-size and larger scaly plaques were scattered over her upper back, chest, arms and face. She began taking high doses of vitamin E daily. Vitamin E was also applied directly to the skin. "After nine months, all lesions were clear," according to the doctors, "except for

A Dermatologist's Best Friend

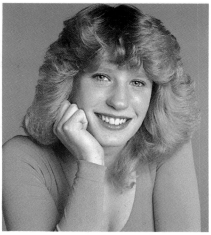

Vitamin E is a great help in achieving beautiful skin, like that of the girl pictured here. But some dermatologists have found that vitamin E also succeeds where all else has failed in clearing up severe dermatological problems.

Consider the case of a 45-year-old man with Raynaud's disease, a circulatory disorder. This man had 6 ulcerated fingers; gangrene actually was present in 3 of them. Yet even this person, whose disease had progressed to a horrendous state, "virtually healed 8 weeks after using vitamin E" both orally and directly on his fingers, reported Samuel Ayres, Jr., M.D., and Richard Mihan, M.D., of Los Angeles. Several other patients with this condition were given vitamin E, and although the results were not as dramatic, the majority showed good progress in healing. Large doses of vitamin E also helped such skin conditions as porphyria cutanea tarda (a metabolism disturbance that causes chronic skin lesions), discoid lupus erythematosus, scleroderma (in which the skin develops pigmented patches) and many other problematic complaints. Dr. Mihan and Dr. Ayres have found that, frequently, good results are not obtained until the dosage of E is well above a few hundred units daily, a level you should take only under a doctor's supervision.

six tiny inconspicuous remnants on the face and left neck."

How does vitamin E accomplish its results? The doctors aren't entirely sure, but they suspect it acts at the cellular level. "Theoretically, vitamin E functions as a first line of defense by protecting cell membranes from destructive lipid peroxidation," they explain. In other words, fatty components in the cell wall may be shielded from harmful oxidation or breakdown when sufficient vitamin E is present.

Vitamin E can also be a protective shield for adults who had chicken pox as children. Unfortunate-

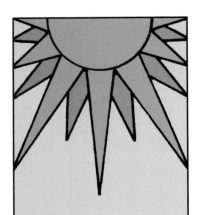

Inside-Out Protection

We now know that *oral* vitamin E may help prevent sunburn, thanks to mice that tanned in the name of science. Hairless mice ate either a plain diet or a diet supplemented with vitamin E and other antioxidants, and then were exposed to sunlamps. The no-E mice suffered "marked erythema" (redness), but the mice taking E did not; in fact, the nutrients *doubled* their sun protection.

ly, the same nasty little bug that gave you chicken pox can come back to haunt you decades later, more severely. The bug: herpes—the disease: shingles. After a bout with chicken pox, herpes zoster (the official name of this virus) sometimes takes up residence in the spinal nerves, where it promptly goes into hibernation. You think it's gone forever, but it can wake up at any time and start multiplying.

When that happens, the affected nerve becomes inflamed and pain radiates all along its path. The herpes virus then passes down the nerve and multiplies again in the skin, causing clusters of sores to erupt.

They start out as small reddened areas, which quickly puff up with fluid to the size of a quarter, or sometimes larger. The skin over the blisters becomes increasingly rigid, until finally by about the fifth day after eruption the blisters burst. During the next week or two, crusts develop, but a total of two to four weeks may elapse before you see the last scab fall off.

All the while you may be feeling extreme discomfort. It's those over age 50 who are most susceptible. And these are not necessarily sickly folks.

Dr. Mihan has treated numerous cases of herpes zoster and the neuralgia (pain that lingers long after the obvious infection has gone) that often accompanies it. Doctors believe the neuralgia is caused by scarring of the damaged nerves. "The pain may be severe at times, requiring sedation and causing almost unbearable discomfort and loss of sleep," says Dr. Mihan. Rather than resorting to drastic measures like cutting out the root of the affected nerve, Dr. Ayres and Dr. Mihan have found a better, safer way to relieve the prolonged suffering. Vitamin E.

Over a period of four years, they treated 13 patients with chronic postherpetic neuralgia with vitamin E, administered both orally and directly on the sores.

Eleven of the patients had had moderate to severe pain for over six months. Seven of those had suffered for over 1 year; one for 13 years and one for 19 years! Yet after taking

vitamin E, nine patients reported complete or almost complete control of pain. The two patients who had had postherpetic neuralgia the longest were in this group. Of the remaining four patients, two were moderately improved and two were slightly improved.

But vitamin E doesn't just relieve pain. It also helps stop the rash from spreading. One woman reported, "I noticed a sore about the size of a silver dollar on my back. When I touched the spot, it burst as if it were a blister. I thought nothing of it until late that same evening when I felt a rash very rapidly spreading all over my back. It was annoying and felt as though ants were crawling on my skin.

"Not knowing how to stop it from spreading, I wondered if vitamin E might help. I cut the tips of three vitamin E capsules (each 400 I.U.) with scissors, let the oil drip into a saucer and applied it to the reddish, tender sores. Vitamin E stopped the rash from spreading instantly and gave me so much relief that I was able to sleep well that night. By morning my husband was amazed to notice how the sores had begun to heal and were already forming scabs.

"I paid a visit to our family doctor that afternoon and he confirmed my own suspicions: It was shingles. Healing progressed quickly and completely as I continued applying vitamin E oil to the infected area, and during that time I was never laid up and was able to do all of my housework. It's no wonder that vitamin E is called the 'miracle vitamin.'"

Natural protection for your circulation, lungs and skin is vitamin E's standard task. But this nutrient's bag of tricks isn't empty yet. It tackles arthritis, cancer and a host of other problems. Let's look at them one by one.

VITAMIN E EASES ARTHRITIS PAIN

In an Israeli study, supplements of vitamin E reduced pain for more than half of a group of people with osteoarthritis.

People Speak on E

There's more to vitamin E than meets the eye that reads only medical literature. Sometimes it's the people actually using the nutrient who provide some of the most insightful information. Consider all these anecdotes about the benefits of using vitamin E to heal skin problems. Remember they reflect personal experiences and are not prescriptions, nor do they carry the same weight as controlled scientific studies. But they do reveal vitamin E's remarkable versatility in healing, both as a last-resort measure and as a "first resort."

"Last August my husband awakened with a rash over his left side. It looked like shingles to me. He went to the doctor that afternoon and sure enough, that's what he had. The doctor said nothing could be done and that my husband would be uncomfortable for several weeks, with burning and itching. I immediately applied vitamin E oil, and continued to do so each morning and night. In 5 days the rash was drying up and he was not uncomfortable at all."

"My 2-year-old son and I went for a hike on the hills and the next day I noticed big red patches and huge whitish welts on his feet, legs and wrists. It was poison oak. I broke open a 400-I.U. vitamin E capsule and applied it to the swollen areas. I gave my son another capsule to swallow. When he arose from his nap an hour later, I was completely astonished. There was not a single trace of the red patches and welts. They'd disappeared!"

"My husband is a diabetic and does not heal very well. He somehow got a boil on his back that grew larger and larger. His doctor said to apply hot packs, and though I did this for 3 months, the boil got larger. Finally I decided to put vitamin E oil on it. In a few days I noticed the boil was becoming smaller. Soon it went away."

"I had a stubborn case of athlete's foot between my little toe and the next one. To my amazement, vitamin E cleared up the problem almost immediately, and there has been no return of the fungus over a 2-month interval."

"The incision from my hip operation was 10 inches long and had 20 stitches. It was quite tender when I came home, and the stitches kept pulling. After 4 uncomfortable days, I turned to vitamin E. I used a 400-I.U. capsule, spreading the contents all over the incision. Wow, what a difference! The stitches no longer pulled and the incision looked much better."

"While on vacation, I noticed a small rough spot on my right side. In a week, it looked very much like a wart. My wife made a pinhole in a vitamin E capsule and dabbed the contents on the wart once a day. In 10 days, it was completely gone."

"When our son came home from a bike trip his shoulders and neck were fiery from sunburn. I 'painted' the burn using several vitamin E capsules. The next morning there was only a crimson patch on his arm where we'd missed."

"My husband severely scalded his right arm with hot water. When he started to wipe the water off, his skin came off with it and he was blistered on other parts of his arm. I applied some burn salve during the first day, but then I remembered that vitamin E eases burns. I immediately broke open the capsules and spread the contents on his arm. In about a week his arm was healed and it left no scar at all."

In the experiment, 29 patients at Hasharon Hospital were randomly assigned to either a group taking 600 I.U. of vitamin E a day or a group taking placebos. Then, after ten days, the groups were switched.

At the end of the experiment, 15 of the 29 "experienced marked relief of pain" while taking vitamin E, while only *1* of the patients had such a reaction to the placebo.

VITAMIN E AND CANCER

Vitamin E's potential as an anticancer agent has just begun to be explored. Researchers at the University of Colorado Health Science Center have found that combinations of vitamin E and anticancer drugs work synergistically, meaning that their combined effect is greater than the sum of their separate abilities.

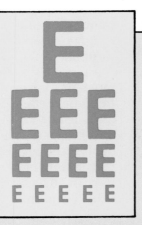

E'ing Is Believing

For diabetics, E stands for eyes—better eyes, that is, with vitamin E. According to some promising research, vitamin E can prevent blood platelets from clumping together—a phenomenon that is associated with the eye disease diabetic retinopathy. In one study, vitamin E was tested on 10 patients with this eye problem and 10 healthy people. Platelet aggregation (clumping) was triggered chemically. When vitamin E was administered, the grouping of platelets slowed in *both* groups. Yet another study, from the University of Western Ontario, suggests the nutrient also may prevent cataracts—particularly cortical cataracts, which occur in the back part of the eye lens. Researchers put rats' lenses in a high-glucose solution and produced a cloudiness similar to that which develops in diabetic cataracts. But adding vitamin E to the solution kept the cataracts from forming.

Ronald R. Watson, Ph.D., at the University of Arizona Health Science Center, has been testing the effects of diet on the immune systems of laboratory animals. "We found that vitamin E boosts one aspect of the immune response, important in the body's anticancer defenses, within a week of giving it to the mice."

Consider also fibrocystic breast disease. Also known as benign cystic mastitis, this disease has certainly frightened many women who have found painful lumps in their breasts. It is responsible for almost three-fourths of all breast surgery—surgery not only to remove the cysts but also to make sure the lumps aren't malignant.

Vitamin E seems to offer a safe, effective remedy for these cysts. At Sinai Hospital in Baltimore, researchers have been using vitamin E successfully in the treatment of cysts for several years. In one experiment, researchers gave 600 I.U. to a group of 26 women every day for two months.

Robert London, M.D., director of the division of clinical research at Sinai Hospital, says, "The cysts cleared up in ten of them. Twelve more had fair responses and only four showed no response to the treatment. That's an overall positive response of 85 percent, and no side effects were noted."

UNCLAMP THAT CRAMP

When a team of Los Angeles doctors gave vitamin E to 125 patients with nighttime leg and foot cramps, 103 had complete or nearly complete relief.

About half of the patients found relief by taking 300 I.U. or less of vitamin E a day. The other half needed 400 I.U. or more to control their cramps. And, the doctors noted, many patients had to continue taking vitamin E to stay free of cramps.

But the doctors treated more than nighttime foot and leg cramps with vitamin E. They also treated cramps from heavy exercise, nighttime rectal cramps and cramping of abdominal muscles.

COOLING HOT FLASHES

Rosetta Reitz, author of *Menopause: A Positive Approach,* believes there is a simple, natural solution to hot flashes.

"Many women," she writes, "have found relief in two days from taking 800 I.U. of vitamin E. I have seen flashes disappear completely when the vitamin E is also accompanied by 2,000 to 3,000 milligrams of vitamin C (taken at intervals throughout the day) and by 1,000 milligrams (also at intervals) of calcium. When the flashes have subsided, usually after a week, the women reduce the vitamin E intake to 400 I.U." (The upper amounts of vitamins C and E that Ms. Reitz suggests should be taken only under a doctor's supervision.)

E FOR INFECTIONS

Overshadowed by vitamin C, vitamin E is an underappreciated source of help for infections, according to an impressive series of studies conducted at Colorado State University. According to Dr. Cheryl Nockels and colleagues in the department of animal sciences at Colorado State University, vitamin E—in amounts well beyond the Recommended Dietary Allowance—can also play a major role in keeping strong the body's defense against infection.

"I tried to determine whether supplements of vitamin E, given in excess of what is required for normal growth and reproduction, increased immunity to infection," she says.

In her experiment, Dr. Nockels and a team of researchers gave one group of mice their normal diet and another a diet supplemented with vitamin E. They injected both groups with sheep red blood cells. Four days later, the mice were examined.

When mice are injected with sheep red blood cells, their bodies react to them the way they'd react to bacteria—by producing the antibodies that take invaders out of action. That vital defense process was significantly stronger in the mice that received the vitamin E.

Straightening the Sickled Cell

Sickle-cell anemia patients have a deficiency of vitamin E, say Danny Chiu, Ph.D., and Bertram Lubin, M.D., of Oakland, California. That lack may contribute to the sickling process, in which red blood cells bend into distorted, crescent shapes. The scientists have found that—at least in the test tube—damage to the red blood cells can be prevented by vitamin E. Dr. Chiu speculates that E's antioxidant effect may alter the red cell membrane's stability, making it less vulnerable to distortion. Still more promising research, from Hoffmann-La Roche Inc. and Columbia University, showed that when 13 patients took 450 I.U. of vitamin E a day, the sickling process slowed: The proportion of their irreversibly sickled cells dropped from 25 to 11 percent.

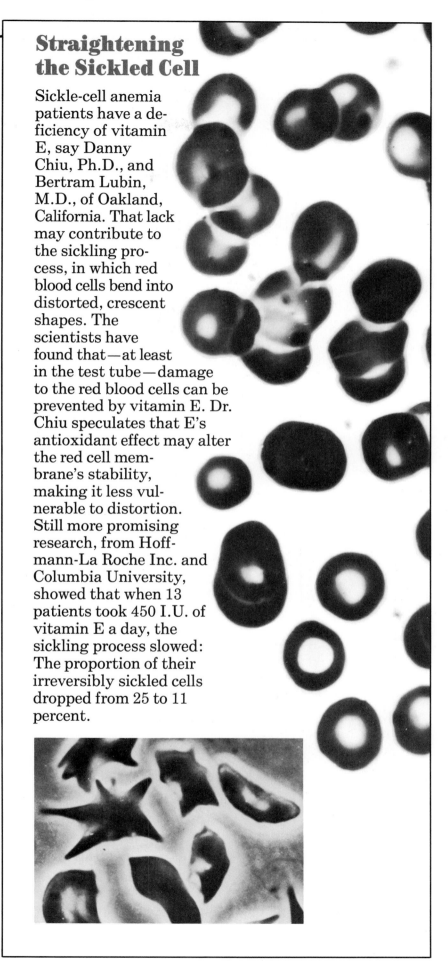

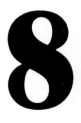

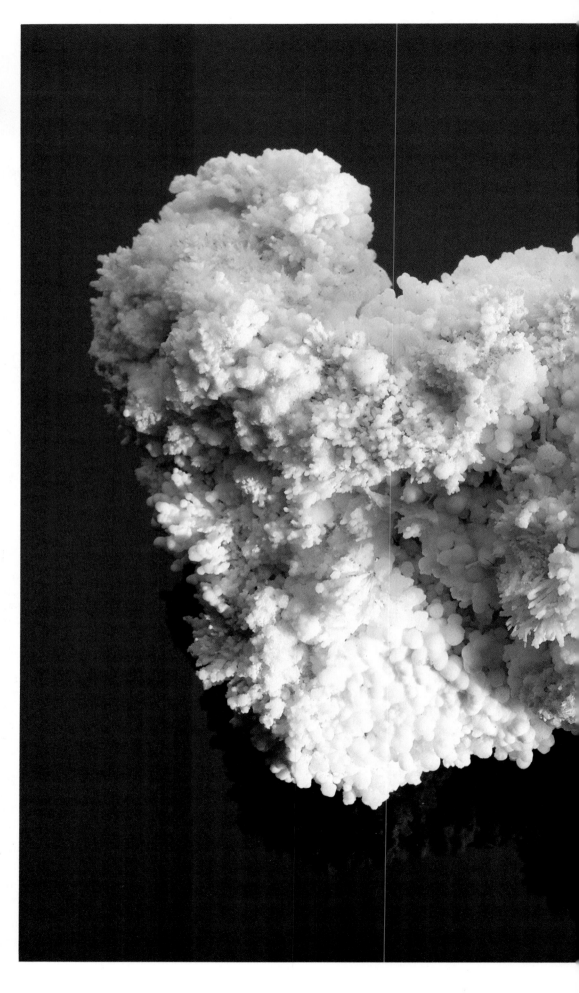

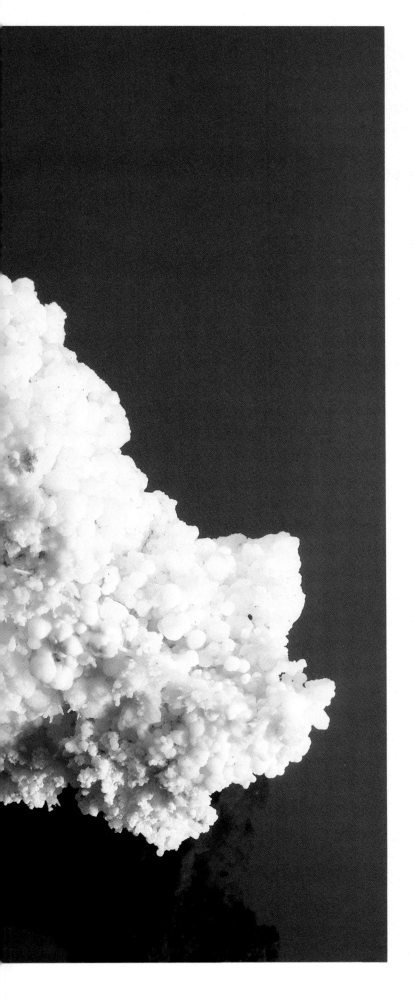

Minerals: Foundation of Health

All the vitamins in the world do us little good without minerals.

"Remember to take your vitamins." It's the last thing many moms and dads say to their kids at breakfast. What parents should say, though, is "Take your vitamins *and* minerals," because minerals like iron and calcium are just as important to health as vitamins A, B complex and the rest of that alphabetical crew.

But even if you know that calcium and iron are good for you, you probably never realized just how good they *really* are. Perhaps you think of iron as an antianemia blood builder. Well, muscles need iron just as much as blood does. And iron helps fight pollution, too. Sure, calcium builds strong bones. But did you know that calcium also helps control blood pressure, clear up depression, relieve menstrual and muscle cramps and guard against heart disease?

And then there are the minerals you've probably never thought twice about—or even heard of—but that you can't do without. The trace mineral selenium, for instance, may be one of the most promising weapons in the nutritional fight against cancer. (Trace, because we need it in only minuscule amounts.) Consider this startling fact: A lower level of selenium in their cigarettes might explain why American, British and Swedish smokers suffer a higher lung cancer rate than smokers in Mexico and Colombia, according to researchers at the New Jersey Medical School. In American, English and Swedish cigarettes, the average selenium content is 0.16 parts per million (ppm), compared to 0.49 ppm in Mexico and Colombia—a significant difference.

Farfetched? Not at all.

"Of all the factors we looked at," says toxicologist John D. Bogden, Ph.D., "selenium was the most likely candidate. A substantial amount of data shows that selenium has anticancer properties."

HEARTENING NEWS

Minerals have also made the news in the area of heart disease research. Six of them—calcium, potassium, magnesium, zinc, chromium and selenium—each help ward off heart disease.

A related problem, high blood pressure, can be controlled by careful attention to calcium, magnesium, potassium and zinc, according to new studies from all over the world.

Zinc and chromium may help control wavering blood sugar levels in diabetics and so reduce—or even possibly eliminate—the need for insulin. In fact, one doctor we know cut his own insulin requirements in half as a result of chromium supplementation. Certainly something to think about if you have blood sugar problems and are planning a personal nutrition program.

In another area of health, modern research has shown that impotence, infertility and prostate troubles may be related to low zinc intake. According to most doctors, there is *no* food or nutrient that can improve—let alone reverse—sexual impotence. Yet a headline in an issue of the medical journal *Sexual Medicine Today* read: "Zinc Supplementation: A New Therapy for Erectile Failure?"

Minerals also help us cope with the special demands of modern life, such as stress and pollution. Studies with animals at the University of Illinois department of animal science showed that even small amounts of zinc protected against lead intake, although larger amounts were better. And similar research has uncovered pollution-protection roles for calcium, magnesium, iron and selenium.

A SHORTER HOSPITAL STAY

Even surgery can go far more smoothly when you've got zinc under your belt. A team of Philadelphia doctors, led by Thomas V. Sedlacek, M.D., used zinc supplements to *cut in half* the number of days women had to remain in the hospital after gynecological surgery. The average postoperative stay for women not receiving zinc supplements was 37

days. But the women who received zinc for a week before their operations were able to go home after just 18 days.

In Dr. Sedlacek's own words, "At current rates, a decrease in hospital stay of this magnitude represents a savings of about $10,000 for each patient. . . ."

What makes the healing power of minerals especially valuable is that they can be a natural, drugless way to treat disease—a way that's not a minefield of side effects. Take a look, for instance, at the use of calcium supplements instead of estrogen to stop bone loss in older women. Estrogen has been linked to breast and uterine cancer, gallbladder disease and high blood pressure—but calcium supplements (in reasonable doses) are 100 percent safe. What's more, calcium can *reverse* bone loss, a claim that estrogen certainly can't make.

Those are only highlights of the breakthroughs occurring in mineral research, yet they prove that minerals deserve equal billing with vitamins.

Trouble is, minerals might not even make it to the audition, because chances are you're slightly deficient in one or more of them.

Studies of calcium intake, for instance, have shown that 75 percent of all women over age 35 get less than the Recommended Dietary Allowance of 800 milligrams a day. That's especially disconcerting when you consider that women need more calcium than anyone else.

THE POTASSIUM RIP-OFF

A diet high in overprocessed foods loads us with extra sodium while starving us of potassium—a ratio that can send blood pressure soaring. To make matters worse, alcohol and caffeinated beverages like coffee, tea and cola flush potassium out of the body. Add it all up, and many people are drastically low in potassium.

You may not be much better off when it comes to magnesium. A study of meals served to students at 50 colleges found that the foods on the menu provided an average of only 251 milligrams of magnesium a day—even though the RDA for magnesium is 350 milligrams for men and 300 for women.

The Nationwide Food Consumption Survey (NFC) found that nearly one-third of the households contacted also served meals that fell short of the daily RDA for magnesium. And approximately one-fifth of the households polled also lacked sufficient iron-rich foods to meet the RDA for that important mineral—10 milligrams for men, 18 milligrams for most women.

Another nationwide survey revealed that 95 percent of American women aged 18 to 44 were getting only a little more than half of the 18 milligrams of iron they need to offset menstrual losses of the mineral. As with calcium, it's a situation in which the people who need iron the most get the least.

Very few Americans, male or female, are getting the amount of zinc they need for optimum health, according to numerous nutritional studies. Researchers who measured the amount of zinc in the diets of elderly people found that most were getting less than two-thirds of the RDA of 15 milligrams. You don't have to be over 60 to be undernourished, though. A similar study of high school girls and college women showed that most of them, too, were getting less than two-thirds of their zinc quota. Other girls in other studies consumed even less than that.

HIGH FAT, LOW CHROMIUM

High levels of sugar and fat in the diet are responsible for a dearth of the trace mineral chromium. One researcher reported that more than half the older people he tested were marginally low in chromium, in spite of the fact that we need only tiny amounts in the first place. Another group of researchers measured the chromium in 14 high-fat diets and found that 8 of them provided less than the recommended intake of chromium.

Selenium is one of the most promising of the health-wielding trace minerals, but here too we tend to lose out. A leading selenium researcher says that the standard diet in this

Are You Low on Arsenic?

In addition to the 7 major minerals discussed in this chapter, a number of less familiar minerals also are essential to health. They are phosphorus, copper, iodine, fluorine, cobalt, sulfur, chlorine and manganese; each one plays a vital and unique role in the body.

Beyond those are even more minerals that occur in trace amounts in our food—and in our bodies—that also are critical to good health. Tin, for instance, stimulates growth in newborns. Certain phases of iron metabolism depend on vanadium. Bones and teeth also need traces of vanadium to grow as they should. Dental enamel is rich in molybdenum, a mineral that seems to share some of fluorine's work in building strong teeth. Molybdenum also functions as part of a special enzyme that liberates iron from the liver. Strontium is similar to calcium in that it helps to build strong bones. Tiny amounts of nickel are not only harmless but essential. Nickel is present in all our tissues and in our blood. It activates enzymes and serves in various body processes.

In addition, it has been shown that barium, bromine and even arsenic are necessary for certain biological reactions. These 3 are among 20 obscure trace minerals now under investigation for their possible contributions to human health and nutrition. Some day, even industrial metals like aluminum and boron or precious metals like gold and silver may prove to affect the "economy" of the human body.

GOLD
TIN
BERYLLIUM
MOLYBDENUM
CESIUM
ALUMINUM
NICKEL
BORON

country skimps on selenium, providing only about 100 micrograms. That's far less than the 200 micrograms needed to fully benefit from the mineral.

The mineral-by-mineral account of these nutrients that follows will show how even slight deficiencies can put you in the gray zone of health—not really sick, but not really well, either. And in some cases, mineral deficiencies directly contribute to major

99

Calcium-Rich Recipe: Tofu Lasagna

Makes 5 servings

4 quarts water
1½ tablespoons oil
½ pound whole wheat
  lasagna noodles
  (about 8 noodles)
1 cup mashed tofu
½ cup grated Parmesan
  cheese

1 egg
½ clove garlic, finely
  minced
1 cup shredded moz-
  zarella cheese
1 cup thinly sliced
  mushrooms

2 tablespoons finely
  chopped fresh
  parsley
2½ cups Basic Tomato
  Sauce *(see
  recipe below)*

In a large pot, bring water to a boil. Add oil to prevent noodles from sticking together as they cook. Add noodles and cook at a rolling boil, stirring occasionally with long wooden fork or spoon, for about 8 minutes, until they are tender. Drain noodles and douse with cold water. Set aside.

While noodles are cooking, mix tofu, ¼ cup Parmesan cheese, egg and garlic. Beat until smooth and fluffy. Have mozzarella, mushrooms and parsley ready for assembly.

Spoon ¼ cup tomato sauce on the bottom of a very lightly greased loaf pan or 1½-quart baking pan. Place 2 noodles on top of sauce. Spread tofu-Parmesan mixture over noodles. Place 2 noodles on top of cheese mixture. Spread mushrooms and parsley over the noodles and add sauce. Place 2 noodles on top and add mozzarella and sauce. Arrange the last noodles and pour remaining sauce over them. Sprinkle with remaining Parmesan cheese. Bake in preheated 350°F oven for 45 to 50 minutes. Allow to stand 5 to 10 minutes before serving.

Basic Tomato Sauce

Makes 2 cups

5 ripe tomatoes, coarsely
  chopped
2 tablespoons olive oil
2 cloves garlic, minced
1¼ cups chopped onions
1 bay leaf
1 teaspoon basil

⅛ teaspoon celery seed
  pinch of thyme
3 sprigs parsley, finely
  chopped
oregano and/or
  cayenne pepper
  to taste

Puree tomatoes in a blender. In a large saucepan, heat oil and saute garlic and onions. Add pureed tomatoes, bay leaf, basil, celery seed and thyme. Cook over low heat for at least 45 minutes (the longer the better.) Add parsley and cook for 2 to 3 minutes more. Remove bay leaf. Season to taste with oregano and/or cayenne.

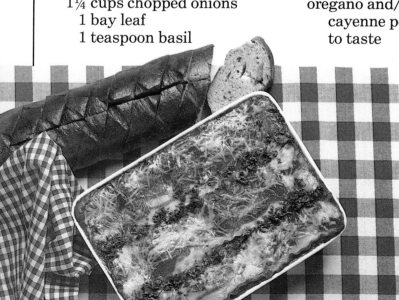

problems like osteoporosis, high blood pressure and diabetes. In other words, vitamins are important—but minerals help create *total* health.

CALCIUM: MORE THAN A BONE BUILDER

We're conditioned to think of calcium in one way and one way only, as a builder of strong bones and teeth. But this is a highly versatile nutrient, playing a wide variety of roles that are crucial to the proper functioning of the body. Calcium is indispensably involved in every beat of our hearts and every thought that passes through our minds.

It's true that 99 percent of the calcium in the body is found in the teeth and bones. Without the work of the other 1 percent, however, life would be impossible.

Calcium is necessary for the proper transmission of messages along the body's nervous system, and at the critical control points where nerves and muscles meet. It plays an important role in muscle contraction, both in relaying the command impulse from nerve to muscle and in the actual contraction of the muscle itself. In fact, if the body does not get enough calcium, the entire neuromuscular system goes haywire.

But even though the muscles and nerves depend on a steady flow of calcium, the mineral's reservoir is in the bones. And too little calcium can turn those reservoirs into crumbling wrecks—a condition called osteoporosis.

In osteoporosis, once-strong bones that could take whatever life dished out become as fragile as china. Porous as a spider's web and as easily broken, they snap at the slightest bump—stepping off a curb, brushing into a table—and often with no bump at all.

Every year *six million* people with osteoporosis—men as well as women—suffer these bone fractures, often spinal fractures that crush the delicate vertebrae, stealing inches from their height and saddling them with a "dowager's hump."

But the bone injury that adds an even worse insult than shrinking

The Best Food Sources of Calcium

Food	Portion	Calcium (mg.)
Swiss cheese	2 oz.	544
Yogurt, skim milk	1 cup	452
Provolone cheese	2 oz.	428
Monterey Jack cheese	2 oz.	424
Cheddar cheese	2 oz.	408
Muenster cheese	2 oz.	406
Colby cheese	2 oz.	388
Brick cheese	2 oz.	382
Sardines, Atlantic, drained solids	3 oz.	371
Mozzarella cheese	2 oz.	366
American cheese	2 oz.	348
Milk, skim	1 cup	302
Buttermilk	1 cup	285
Limburger cheese	2 oz.	282
Salmon, sockeye, drained solids	3 oz.	274
Broccoli, cooked	1 medium stalk	158
Dandelion greens, cooked	½ cup	147
Pizza, cheese	⅛ of a 14-in. pie	144
Blackstrap molasses	1 tbsp.	137
Soy flour	½ cup	132
Collards, cooked	½ cup	110
Tofu	3 oz.	109
Kale, cooked	½ cup	103

is a hip fracture. One out of every six people who have a hip fracture because of osteoporosis dies within three months, literally wasting away in a hospital bed.

Why are postmenopausal women singled out as the most likely victims of this disease—with 90 percent of all postmenopausal women losing a significant amount of bone tissue?

Because at menopause the production of the female hormone estrogen slows down. And while estrogen controls the menstrual cycle, it also acts to hold calcium in the bones. With less estrogen, calcium trickles out of the bones in a steady, year-after-year flow until, shrunken and weak, they collapse.

Some doctors have tried to solve this problem by giving women either calcium or estrogen. In a study comparing these two treatments, 61

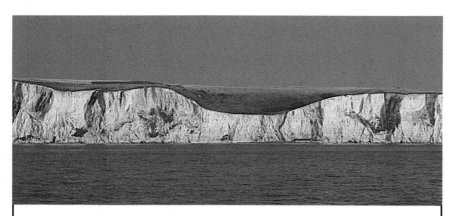

What about Bone Meal and Dolomite?

A few years ago, lead was detected in samples of bone meal and dolomite (which is found in the White Cliffs of Dover, shown above), raising questions about the safety of these calcium supplements. Bone meal samples subsequently tested by the FDA averaged 4.4 ppm of lead, which means 3 teaspoons of bone meal containing 5 ppm of lead would give you 50 micrograms of the mineral. (The minimum "safe" limits for total lead intake are 100 micrograms a day for infants, 150 for children and 429 for adults, a certain amount of lead being unavoidable). Rodale Press employed a laboratory to test dolomite and found that none of the samples contained more than the equivalent of 7 micrograms to 3 average tablets—far less than even bone meal.

Still, some people worry that *any* lead may be harmful. If you are one of them, you can rely on other calcium compounds with total confidence, such as calcium gluconate and calcium carbonate.

One problem. Cancer.

Surveys have shown a definite relationship between estrogen use and endometrial (uterine) cancer.

"From 1940, the incidence of endometrial cancer in the United States was more or less stable, but a marked rise was noted for the period 1969 to 1973 in data from a number of cancer registries," said a study published in the *Lancet,* a medical journal. "This rise exceeded 10 percent per year in some areas and was greatest in women aged 45 to 74 years. It was suggested the increase might relate to use of estrogens, sales of which have risen fourfold in the years 1963-73." And, the study continued, "a fall in estrogen prescriptions in early 1976 was followed by a fall, within a year, in endometrial cancer incidence."

Besides cancer of the uterus, estrogen therapy has been linked to breast cancer, gallbladder disease, high blood pressure, breast tenderness and other ailments.

So forget about estrogen.

Calcium is the better way, and striking new findings at Hammersmith Hospital in London have added confirmation to that fact. In a study that involved tracking 48 osteoporosis patients over a period of ten years (an average 3½ years of participation by each patient), a team of endocrinologists think they may have found the best proof yet that calcium by itself can reverse osteoporosis—and do it effectively for long periods of time.

The patients were divided into two groups. The first group included 25 people who suffered from "typical" osteoporosis—24 postmenopausal women and one man over 60. Their average age was 67. The second group included 23 men and women suffering from osteoporosis for other, less common reasons. Their average age was 47.

The study was organized in four stages. In the initial stage, the patients were put on calcium lactate gluconate supplements according to their individual needs. They continued taking calcium supplements throughout the experiment. In the second stage, the patients were given a hormonal regimen and in the third stage they were switched to another

postmenopausal women were divided into three groups. One group received no treatment, another group got 800 milligrams of calcium, and the third received estrogen. The size of their bones was measured when the study began and again two years later.

"The untreated group continued to lose bone during the two years," reported the researchers, while "the estrogen group lost none." Those in the calcium-treated group lost some bone mass, but far less than the untreated group.

Fine, you say. Lead me to the estrogen and a life long on both years and bones.

hormonal regimen. At stage four, all hormone therapy was stopped.

At each stage, patients were tested for their "calcium balance." Calcium balance simply means the difference between the amount of calcium going into the body and the amount being excreted. At the end of the study their calcium balances were measured for the last time.

The experiment was a success in terms of nutrition and health. It showed that each patient's calcium balance improved and that more calcium was returning to jeopardized bones and making them stronger. The removal of the hormones at stages three and four lowered the calcium balance, but overall it still remained positive.

For the researchers, this meant that calcium, as well as being safe, is apparently effective for all but the most stubborn cases of osteoporosis. They concluded, "We consider that the first line of treatment for most osteoporotic patients is to institute a high calcium intake and to reserve supplementary hormone treatment for those patients with continuing vertebral fractures, occurring, say, after a year on high calcium alone."

Some doctors are also investigating calcium in combination with vitamin D, which helps the body absorb more of the dietary calcium. One of these is Ashok Vaswani, M.D., of the Brookhaven National Laboratory, who believes that the right amount of supplemental calcium for most people is 1,000 to 1,500 milligrams per day.

Patrick Ober, M.D., an endocrinologist at the Bowman Gray School of Medicine, Winston-Salem, North Carolina, also uses calcium and vitamin D instead of estrogen.

"When there are two kinds of treatments, and one, like calcium, is benign and just as effective, then I'm inclined to go with it," he explains. "There doesn't seem to be any hazard to taking calcium."

James Buchanan, M.D., of Pennsylvania State University, has treated osteoporosis patients with a daily combination of 1,000 milligrams of calcium and a very small amount of a synthetic, more potent form of vitamin D. "I feel like I've got a good thing going here, with a low risk,"

Calcium: The Best Denture Adhesive

For most people who've lost their natural teeth, wearing dentures is one continuous hassle. Even the best false teeth are clumsy and irritating.

A big part of the problem is the bony ridge on which dentures are supposedly anchored.

"In a great percentage of denture wearers, the jawbone keeps shrinking away," says Kenneth E. Wical, D.D.S., chairman of the removable prosthetics department of Loma Linda University's School of Dentistry. "As the jawbone grows smaller, it becomes more difficult for people to wear dentures."

Extra calcium can slow that process down, making dentures more bearable. Dr. Wical studied 2 groups of denture wearers—one group took 750 milligrams of calcium (plus vitamin D); the other did not. At the end of 1 year, the people taking extra calcium lost an average of 34 percent less jawbone than the others, leaving them with a firmer hold on their dentures.

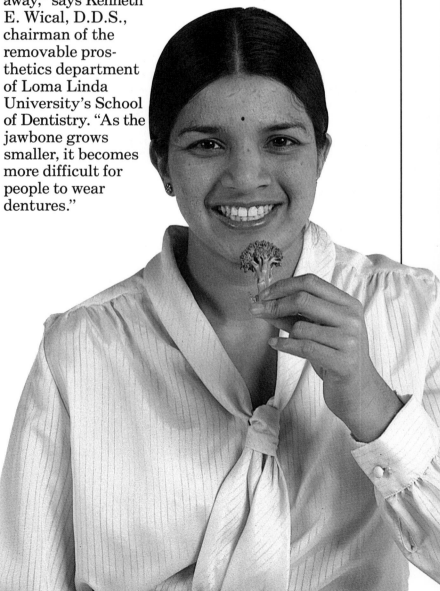

he says. "Estrogen works, but there's no reason to use it as long as the calcium/vitamin D combination works."

Dr. Buchanan treated about 150 patients in a two-year period. Many of them were unable to walk, lie down, or do something as simple as sewing, without pain. He was able to relieve pain and disability in 85 percent of the patients. He says he gets results in a few months.

BONE PAIN RELIEVED

Calcium also offers hope for victims of Paget's disease, a type of bone degeneration that's less common than osteoporosis, but sometimes far more painful—deep, dull, aching bone pain is one of the symptoms. Doctors don't know what causes Paget's disease, although it sometimes runs in families. Any bone in the body may be affected, but the most common sites are the long bones of the legs, the lower spine, the pelvis and the skull. In the early stages of the disease, calcium is removed from the bones, softening them. In later stages, the bones begin to grow again. But, somehow, the new growth is distorted. The bones remain soft and become abnormally thick.

Until a few years ago, there was no effective treatment for Paget's disease, although doctors tried several drugs and therapies. Then it was discovered that calcitonin, a hormone secreted by the thyroid gland, relieved pain when given by injection. Unfortunately, the treatment is expensive. The drug also produces nausea in many people, and may be the cause of allergic reactions.

But a safe, effective, low-cost treatment for Paget's disease has been developed by an Australian physician. Dr. R. A. Evans, Repatriation General Hospital, Concord, New South Wales, successfully used calcium supplements and a combination of medications designed to keep blood levels of calcium high in nine patients with Paget's disease. In his study, Dr. Evans gave the patients from 500 to 1,000 milligrams of calcium three times a day between meals, an antacid tablet with meals to keep phosphorus from interfering with calcium absorption and a drug to keep calcium from being excreted in the urine. The treatment continued for 200 days.

In Dr. Evans's words, "Bone pain subsided or was considerably reduced in eight of the nine patients after a period of 20 to 70 days. . . . Two female patients who were invalids prior to commencing therapy were able to return to light household duties. There were no serious side effects."

Dr. Evans believes the treatment works by stimulating the thyroid gland's natural secretion of calcitonin, which occurs when blood levels of calcium rise. Biochemical tests performed by Dr. Evans confirmed that his patients were not merely experiencing a "placebo response" to the treatment.

Dr. Evans goes on to say that "The regimen described here costs

Calcium Quiets Cramps

Two doctors we know treat muscle cramps with calcium.

"For muscle contraction to be normal, adequate levels of calcium must be present in the body," says Ralph Smiley, M.D., of Dallas, Texas. "We make sure that all our patients with cramps are getting enough calcium."

For mild cases of cramps, Dr. Smiley prescribes 900 milligrams of calcium a day. William Rea, M.D., his associate, has also treated hundreds of cramp patients with calcium.

"All these patients had low levels of calcium," Dr. Rea says.

In a survey that *Prevention* magazine conducted to find out the many ways calcium can improve health, more than half the people who replied said that calcium relieves muscle spasms or cramps. Here's a typical comment:

"I had cramps sometimes going from my little finger up to my shoulder and all the way down my spine. After taking 1,800 milligrams of calcium daily, all the cramps were completely eliminated."

approximately 2 percent [of the cost of the usual drug treatment] and can be made still cheaper by the use of simpler forms of the drugs. . . . In view of the extremely low cost of this drug combination and its lack of side effects, it is suggested it be considered as a treatment for Paget's disease of bone."

AN END TO GUM DISEASE

Periodontal (gum) disease is another manifestation of calcium deficiency. And in a sense, gum disease and the jawbone deterioration that usually goes with it are actually a manifestation of osteoporosis. And periodontal disease is the leading cause of tooth loss in adults.

Fortunately, calcium can help save your gums and teeth while it's saving your bones. In a study performed at Cornell University by Lennart Krook, D.V.M., Ph.D., Leo Lutwak, M.D., and other doctors, five men and five women with advanced periodontal disease were given 500 milligrams of calcium twice a day over a period of six months.

"All patients had gingivitis [gum inflammation] and bleeding at the start," the researchers reported. "After treatment, inflammation was improved in all cases and absent in three." The doctors noticed other benefits as well. Pockets at the gum line were reduced, and previously loose and wobbly teeth tended to tighten up in their sockets. The jawbones—which had been losing mineral density before—began to re-form and lay down new bone growth.

CALMING CALCIUM

"A tiny decrease of calcium in the blood can produce uncontrollable temper outbursts," warn Emanuel Cheraskin, M.D., D.M.D., and W. Marshall Ringsdorf, Jr., D.M.D., of the department of oral medicine at the University of Alabama in Birmingham.

And that can happen, especially during times of sudden, unexpected emotional stress. That's because at those times the blood lactic acid

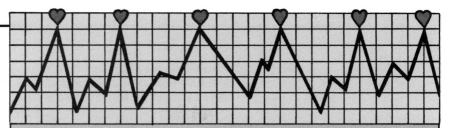

Your Heart Loves Calcium

Researchers have found that supplemental calcium can lessen the amount of cholesterol clogging up your arteries.

Harold Yacowitz, Ph.D., at Fairleigh Dickinson University in Madison, New Jersey, found that 1,600 milligrams of total calcium a day lowered cholesterol by 48 points and triglycerides by 115 points in people he studied.

Marvin L. Bierenbaum, M.D., at St. Vincent's Hospital in Montclair, New Jersey, gave 2,000 milligrams of dietary calcium a day to 10 people with high blood fats. After a year, their cholesterol

dropped by 25 percent.

Calcium helps your heart by reducing the consequence of cholesterol: arterial plaque, which forms when cholesterol hardens on the lining of the arteries. If cholesterol is allowed to line your arteries, they'll harden, making your heart work harder. In addition to reducing cholesterol, calcium also fights heart disease by lowering blood pressure. Researchers at Oregon Health Sciences University found that calcium intake in people with normal blood pressure was significantly higher than in those with high blood pressure.

levels can rise considerably, which has the effect of depleting circulating calcium. The result is a lot of anxiety or a volatile temper.

But calcium supplements or a calcium-rich diet can restore blood levels to normal and smooth out jagged nerves.

In fact, calcium supplements of various kinds alleviated an array of related health problems for many of the thousands of people who responded to a survey conducted by *Prevention* magazine. Over half the respondents —1,653, to be exact—said that taking extra calcium relieved muscle spasms or cramps. For example, a woman from Houston, Texas, reported that calcium relieved cramping in her calves. At age 60, she said, she retired from nursing and went into sales. She had to stand on hard floors for long hours, causing a great deal of pain and cramping in her legs at night. She began to take one dolomite tablet before each meal and another at bedtime, which in her words, "has made a new woman out of me."

An impressive number of people —1,379—said that calcium relieved bone pain. Another 1,304 said calcium helped their nerves or made them less irritable and 1,010 reported that calcium relieved dental discomforts. Circulation improved for another 495.

Improvement or total relief of menstrual cramping and distress was reported by 293 women—about 10 percent of the total. A woman from Phoenix, Arizona, remarked that "For ten years I took birth control pills to avoid the terrible menstrual cramps that sent me to bed every month since I began to menstruate. But I was afraid of the Pill, so I tried calcium. Now I have absolutely no incapacitating menstrual cramps."

Insomnia, too, disappeared for 256 people who took calcium. An individual from Berkeley, California, wrote that "I can remember even as a very small child being up most of the middle hours of the night. My sleep has always been sort of a state of semiconsciousness. It has caused me a great deal of grief and made it very hard to work at jobs that required fixed hours.

"Now," she continued, "insomnia has become a thing of the past—this has totally changed my life. I take one calcium pill before bed. If I wake up in the middle of the night, I take another. Within half an hour, I'm asleep."

The people who were the most overjoyed, though, were those who experienced less arthritis pain.

"My health was always good, except for arthritis of the hip of five years' duration, with agonizing gnawing pain," said a woman from Hendersonville, North Carolina. "Much of that time I had to walk with a cane, could not carry anything heavy and literally crawled up stairs, holding on to the banisters with both hands.

"I was told by the M.D.'s that I'd have to learn to live with it. After six months of calcium, the pain vanished completely, and has not returned. My health is excellent—my back's straight and very strong, and I can *run* up stairs."

Clearly, the benefits of calcium go well beyond building strong bones to strengthen and repair nearly every part of the body.

How do you make sure you're getting enough calcium? If you were to depend on milk, you'd have to drink at least three glasses a day along with your meals to get "bone-a-fide" protection. But those three glasses are packed with calories and fat. So you should make a habit of including other dairy products like skim milk and buttermilk, which are equally rich in calcium but have fewer calories. Good nondairy sources of calcium are salmon (canned with bones), sardines (canned with bones), soybeans, tempeh, tofu, filberts, almonds, broccoli and dark green, leafy vegetables (collard, turnip and mustard greens and kale).

Still, dozens of dietary surveys and studies have shown that very few people—especially women—get as much calcium as they ought to.

Worse, health scientists have shown that even if the Recommended Dietary Allowance of 800 milligrams a day of calcium *is* met, that isn't enough for many women. A truly protective amount is believed to be somewhere between 1,000 and 1,500 milligrams a day. Many diets, however, fail to provide half that much. The bones get weaker, taking millions of people one step closer to all the problems of calcium deficiency.

To ensure that you're getting enough calcium every day, keep a diet diary for a week, and add up the milligrams of calcium you consumed. (See the chart on page 101 for some common foods and their calcium content.)

GETTING ENOUGH MEANS GETTING *MORE* THAN THE RDA

There's no guesswork going on here, either. Studies were done at major universities to determine what the exact daily intake of calcium should be. To do that, researchers set up a controlled environment for volunteers. These people actually lived in a metabolic-study ward for months at a time. In that way the researchers could measure the precise amount of calcium intake and the exact amount being excreted. The studies showed that for a woman to achieve perfect calcium balance she needs to consume at least 1,300 milligrams per day. That's 500 milligrams more than the RDA. Unfortunately, more than half the women in America ingest 500 milligrams or less of calcium per day.

And doctors suggest even more calcium for postmenopausal women. Robert Recker, M.D., a researcher from Creighton University in Omaha, and his colleagues have published data suggesting that for those women the RDA for calcium should be raised to 1,500 milligrams. But he's also quick to warn other women not to neglect their calcium needs when dieting, pregnant or lactating.

For extra safety, you might want to take a calcium supplement of at least 500 milligrams a day. And although we've been talking mostly about women's health, men would be wise to get enough calcium, too. (Remember, it helps protect against heart attacks.)

POTASSIUM FOR HIGH BLOOD PRESSURE

Potassium performs countless vital functions in the body. It helps nerves transmit messages, aids digestive enzymes in their work, guides normal growth and serves as an electrolyte (that is, it carries a tiny electrical charge that ensures the proper functioning of every muscle in the body, most notably the heart muscle). In certain cases, low potassium may lead to sudden death.

But in its missions, potassium is intimately and mysteriously linked to the activities of sodium. The two substances carry on a sort of unceasing tug-of-war across the walls of the cells. At stake is the delicate electrical and chemical balance of the body.

The Best Food Sources of Potassium

Food	Portion	Potassium (mg.)
Potato	1 medium	782
Avocado	½ medium	602
Raisins	½ cup	545
Sardines, Atlantic, drained solids	3 oz.	501
Flounder	3 oz.	498
Orange juice	1 cup	496
Squash, winter	½ cup	473
Banana	1 medium	451
Apricots, dried	¼ cup	448
Tomato, raw	1 medium	444
Milk, skim	1 cup	406
Salmon, fillet, fresh, cooked	3 oz.	378
Great Northern beans, cooked	½ cup	374
Buttermilk	1 cup	371
Milk, whole	1 cup	370
Cod	3 oz.	345
Sweet potato	1 medium	342
Beef liver	3 oz.	323
Apricots, fresh	3 medium	313
Peach	1 medium	308
Round steak, trimmed of fat	3 oz.	298
Haddock	3 oz.	297
Pork, trimmed of fat	3 oz.	283
Leg of lamb, trimmed of fat	3 oz.	274
Turkey, white meat	3 oz.	259
Turkey, dark meat	3 oz.	247
Tuna, drained solids	3 oz.	225
Chicken, white meat	3 oz.	201

When sodium is winning, the cells contain more water, and potassium is dumped into the urine for excretion. When potassium is winning, the cells get rid of sodium and water. Though sodium has its own role to play in the body's chemistry, it is needed only in minute amounts—and anything above that can be considered a potassium burglar, robbing the system of a vital mineral and sending it on its way where it will do nobody any good.

Various studies of this cellular shoot-out have turned up intriguing new indications that potassium may somehow act as a shield against sodium-induced high blood pressure. In one study, a group of 16 people with mild hypertension and a group with normal blood pressure received two different diets, each for a period of 12 weeks. During the first 12 weeks, both groups ate their normal diet, plus sodium tablets. During the second period, their normal diets were supplemented with potassium, and they were instructed to avoid excessively salty foods and not to add salt while cooking or at the

The high-sodium diet produced a slow rise in blood pressure in both groups. But during the high-potassium/low-sodium diet, "both systolic and diastolic blood pressure fell sharply and significantly in the hypertensive group in contrast to small, but insignificant rises in the normotensive [healthy] group,"

according to the researchers.

A month after the study had ended and the people had returned to their regular eating habits, both groups were tested one final time. It was discovered that the hypertensives' blood pressure had shot right back up again. The researchers concluded that the key factor in the startling drop in pressure during the high-potassium/low-sodium diet had been the increased potassium, since their regular diets included only a marginal rise in sodium but a much greater decline in potassium.

"We'd probably see some dramatic changes in the incidence of hypertension if Americans cut their salt intake to less than 3 grams a day and started eating an equivalent amount of potassium," says Harold B. Battarbee, Ph.D., an associate professor of physiology at Louisiana State University School of Medicine in Shreveport. Dr. Battarbee and pharmacology professor John W. Dailey, Ph.D., searching for some hormonal "missing link" between salt and high blood pressure, discovered that when rats were fed enough salt to make them hypertensive, the levels of two adrenal hormones went down. But doubling the rats' potassium intake prevented the decline—and also significantly slowed the rise in blood pressure.

Curious about how the sodium/potassium balance might affect people with a family history of hypertension, researchers at London Hospital Medical College set up a study in which they altered the two nutrients in the diets of two groups of young men, one with and one without a family history of high blood pressure. They discovered that, in both groups, sodium loading in the diet caused a "similar and insignificant" increase in blood pressure, much like in the first experiment. But when dietary potassium levels were increased at the same time sodium was reduced, the researchers noted a "striking contrast" in the responses of the two groups.

Among the sons of normotensive parents, potassium had no effect or slightly raised the blood pressure, while among those with hypertension in the family, it significantly lowered the pressure.

An Orange instead of Salt Tablets

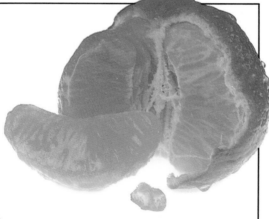

Here's a widely held misconception about heat: If you sweat a lot, you lose so much sodium that you'll get sick; to replace it, you must take salt tablets.

First of all, our bodies acclimate to heat, automatically conserving sodium. The only people who even remotely might need salt tablets are athletes competing in a hot climate for the first time. Even then, sodium would be given only on a doctor's say-so.

Potassium, however, *is* lost during a heat wave, making you feel tired and uncomfortable. During the next hot spell, forget the sodium and instead boost your intake of high-potassium foods. An orange, for instance, contains 263 milligrams of the mineral.

Perhaps, the scientists suggested, it is only those who have a family history of high blood pressure who are sensitive to the pressure-lowering effects of potassium, and they may actually develop hypertension if the potassium level in their diet is inadequate.

Yet other studies seem to suggest that potassium's gentle powers have an effect on nearly everybody, even those without the family curse. In one survey, 86 vegetarian Seventh-Day Adventists were compared with 86 nonvegetarian Mormons (both groups abstain from alcohol, nicotine and caffeine). Writing in *Preventive Medicine,* the researchers noted that it was discovered that "both groups have lower than average blood pressure, but vegetarians had significantly lower blood pressure than did nonvegetarians."

Since fresh fruits and vegetables are among the best sources of potassium, could it be that increased reliance on them results in a higher potassium/sodium ratio and thereby acts as a natural high blood pressure preventive?

That conclusion is suggested by a study conducted in Evans County, Georgia. A dietary analysis of random samples of the white and black populations revealed that although there was no real difference in sodium intake between whites and blacks, the blacks consumed less than half the amount of potassium that whites did—and their blood pressure, as a group, was also considerably higher. (Nationwide, hypertension is almost twice as common among blacks as among whites; the reason is a matter of dispute.)

The researchers concluded that "the only way to explain the higher prevalence of hypertension among blacks appears to be their much lower potassium intake, caused by low consumption of fresh fruit, salads, vegetables, and the traditional long cooking of meats and vegetables with loss of intracellular potassium into the cooking water."

But it's not just good old Southern cookin' that's the problem. Dr. Battarbee points out that resisting civilization's processed foods would help normal pressure stay normal.

Why? Because potassium is substantially lost when foods are canned or frozen. Not only that, but the natural balance between sodium and potassium is actually reversed. According to the USDA's *Nutritive Value of American Foods in Common Units,* Handbook No. 456, for example, a cup of raw peas contains 458 milligrams of potassium and just 3 milligrams of sodium. But when those same peas are canned, salt added during the process raises the sodium level to 588 milligrams (a nearly 200-fold increase), while the potassium is roughly halved, down to 239 milligrams. That's to say nothing about what happens to the proportions when the peas hit the dinner table dressed in table salt and salted butter!

No minimum daily requirement for potassium has been established by the National Research Council, though 2.5 grams (2,500 milligrams) is the commonly cited figure, with a safe range between 2 and 6 grams a day. Sodium, by contrast, is required in only tiny amounts, with half a gram a day or even less usually considered sufficient to fulfill its bodily role. (One teaspoon of salt contains a shade more than 2 grams of sodium.)

Dr. Battarbee admits he doesn't know the ideal ratio of potassium to sodium, but "keeping it to 1 to 1 would be beneficial, though that doesn't mean it's optimal . . . less sodium would be better." Author and chemist Philip S. Chen, Ph.D., claims the ratio should be closer to 2 to 1.

Compare that to the estimated daily intake of the average North American, who gets about 3 grams of salt naturally from his food, another 4 to 6 added during commercial processing, plus 3 added by the cook and at the table. That comes to something like 10 or 12 grams of salt a day (about 4 or 5 grams of sodium). At the same time, we've seen that potassium is often depleted in processed foods.

What's good for your blood pressure is good for your heart—in more ways than one.

Cardiac muscle appears extremely sensitive to potassium content. Sudden

Diuretics Drain Potassium

Diuretic drugs, widely prescribed for high blood pressure, flush potassium out of the body. When that happens, you're in double jeopardy, because potassium is one of the minerals you need to keep blood pressure under control.

How can you escape a potassium leak? By eating plenty of lean meats, fruits like dried apricots and cantaloupe and vegetables like lima beans and potatoes. All are brimming with the mineral. Also see the chart on page 107 for a list of foods high in potassium.

drops in potassium can cause cardiac arrhythmias to occur. Those increased and irregular heartbeats can bring the heart's work to an abrupt and fatal halt.

ENERGY LEVELS IMPROVE WITH POTASSIUM

Your heart isn't the only muscle that demands potassium. Even a slight deficit can sap all your muscles of strength—leaving you tired, weak and irritable. In a study published in the *Journal of the American Medical Association*, researchers randomly selected a group of people and measured their potassium intake. Those people with a deficient intake of potassium—60 percent of the men and 40 percent of the women in the study—had a weaker grip than those with a normal intake. And as potassium intake decreased, muscular strength decreased.

After a few weeks of that kind of weakness and fatigue, you can end up feeling totally dragged out.

"In chronic potassium deficit," according to a researcher who stud-ied potassium, "muscular weakness may persist for many months and be interpreted as being due to emotional disability."

So the sooner you get back to a potassium-rich diet, the more energetic you'll feel.

BEAT THE HEAT

Summer is by far the most critical time for potassium intake. During a heat wave, you need potassium the *most* but are likely to get the *least* from your diet.

During a two-week July hot spell in Detroit, Stanley H. Schuman, M.D., and George W. Williams, Ph.D., of the University of Michigan School of Public Health, measured the effects of heat stress on the body's potassium supply in 631 university hospital outpatients. They described the hot spell as "warm but not record breaking." During the first week, humidity was stifling, with average daytime temperatures in the eighties and average nighttime readings in the sixties. During the second week, daytime highs climbed into the nineties for four straight days. All told, 115 "excess" deaths in the city were reported during the heat wave.

Did low potassium levels have something to do with those deaths? After running more than a dozen biochemical tests on the volunteers, the researchers compared the results with similar readings taken on 698 outpatients at the same hospital during a cool two-week period a month earlier.

Dr. Schuman and Dr. Williams discovered a drop in potassium levels from June to July. Although the dip was not enough to count as an outright deficiency, they described it as "significantly lower."

The researchers speculated the reason for that drop was the potassium-poor meals many people eat in summer. "The inclination to substitute fad foods such as carbonated beverages, alcoholic drinks, low-calorie substitutes and convenient snacks instead of balanced meals is probably never stronger than during the malaise, fatigue and discomfort of sustained humid hot weather,"

Scientists subjected 6 groups of rats to "noise stress" for 3 months. The stress robbed their bodies of magnesium—and the louder the noise, the greater the decrease in magnesium levels. In tests on people (who had to listen to loud traffic noise for 8 hours), results were the same. That means if you live or work where it's noisy, chances are you need extra magnesium.

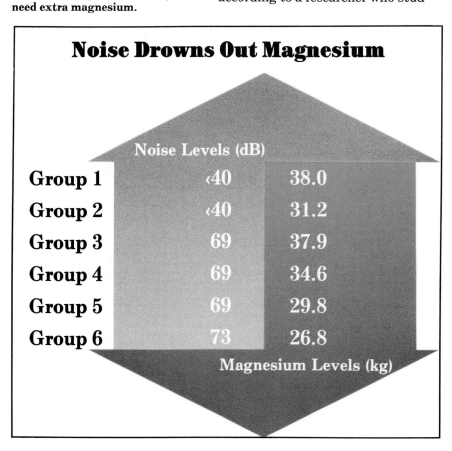

Noise Drowns Out Magnesium

	Noise Levels (dB)	Magnesium Levels (kg)
Group 1	‹40	38.0
Group 2	‹40	31.2
Group 3	69	37.9
Group 4	69	34.6
Group 5	69	29.8
Group 6	73	26.8

wrote the researchers. Unfortunately, such items are exactly the ones most likely to be lacking in potassium.

It's a good idea, therefore, to take advantage of the summer's bounty and eat lots of fresh salad greens, vegetables and fruits—all excellent sources of potassium.

Dr. Schuman and Dr. Williams concluded their study, reported in *Ecology of Food and Nutrition,* with this carefully worded suggestion: "... improvements in dietary intake during hot weather might reduce some morbidity and mortality associated with recent urban heat waves ... it may be prudent during prolonged hot spells to advise heat-susceptible segments of the population to watch the potassium values of foods consumed and for their physicians to be alert for early and reversible signs of potassium depletion."

MAGNESIUM WORKS WONDERS

Many people are first introduced to magnesium in high school chemistry class. In what's known as a "flame test," various metals are heated to their burning point, producing characteristic colors. Magnesium burns with a starlike brilliance that lights up the entire lab. And you need the mineral in your diet to give your body that same kind of radiant, healthy shine.

Magnesium occurs in large amounts in a wide variety of foods. Yet, as we noted earlier, nearly one-third of the households surveyed in one study fell short of the RDA for magnesium. When you realize just how many ways your body depends on magnesium, that statistic is cause for concern.

There is an increasing amount of evidence that many sudden heart failures among "Type A" young men—those who maintain a constant state of self-induced stress—might be due to magnesium deficiency.

In a major report published by the National Research Council of Canada, researchers listed a variety of possible causes of magnesium deficiency and a variety of illnesses that this deficiency might cause. In one study, they noted, the hearts of cardiac victims contained about 22

The Best Food Sources of Magnesium

Food	Portion	Magnesium (mg.)
Soy flour	½ cup	155
Soybeans, dried	¼ cup	138
Buckwheat flour, light	½ cup	112
Black-eyed peas, dried, cooked	¼ cup	98
Almonds, whole	¼ cup	96
Tofu	3 oz.	95
Cashews	¼ cup	94
Kidney beans, dried, cooked	¼ cup	82
Lima beans, dried, raw	¼ cup	81
Brazil nuts	¼ cup	79
Pecans, halved	¼ cup	77
Whole wheat flour	½ cup	68
Shredded wheat	1 cup	67
Peanuts, roasted, chopped	¼ cup	63
Walnuts, black, chopped	¼ cup	60
Banana	1 medium	58
Beet greens, raw, chopped	1 cup	58
Avocado	½ medium	56
Peanut butter	2 tbsp.	56
Peanut flour	¼ cup	54
Blackstrap molasses	1 tbsp.	52
Potato	1 medium	51
Oatmeal	1 cup	50

percent less magnesium than the hearts of those who died of noncardiac problems. And the magnesium shortage was most acute where the heart muscle was infarcted: destroyed due to ischemia, or choked-off blood circulation.

Stress has also been shown to play a role in the SDIHD syndrome—sudden death ischemic heart disease, or sudden heart failure. Magnesium specialist Bella T. Altura, Ph.D., of the State University of New York's Downstate Medical Center in Brooklyn, believes there is a close link among stress, magnesium deficiency and SDIHD. She has found that stress indirectly causes the body to excrete magnesium, resulting in a magnesium deficiency in the heart muscle.

The theory, as developed by Dr. Altura, her husband, Burton M.

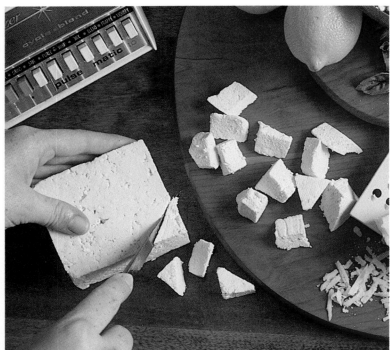

Tofu, a cheeselike food made from soybeans, is one of the richest sources of magnesium—and one of the most versatile. Shown here is one way to use tofu; it is cubed, then creamed in a blender for use in a party spread.

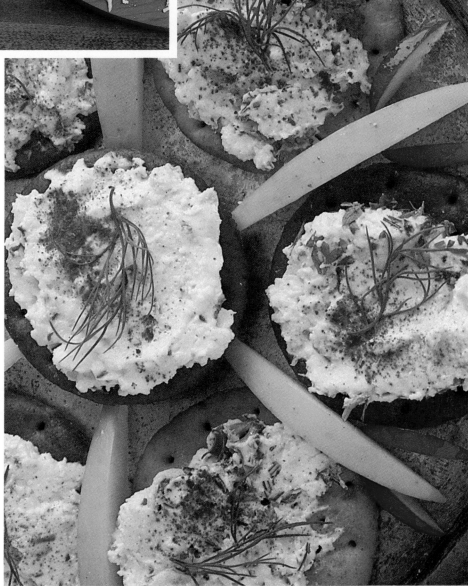

Altura, Ph.D., and Prasad Turlapaty, Ph.D., is this: Magnesium is required for dilating (opening) the blood vessels in the heart tissues, and calcium is required for constricting (closing) the vessels. A delicate balance of magnesium and calcium keeps the heart beating smoothly. A shortage of magnesium means an imbalance toward constriction. A blood vessel may go into spasm and contract suddenly, cutting off circulation to a section of the heart and inducing heart failure.

One of the earliest clues was the observation that the incidence of SDIHD is highest in areas where the drinking water or the soil contains only small amounts of magnesium.

Finland, for example, has one of the highest SDIHD rates of any country in the world; there are also distinct differences in mortality rates from region to region. Studies of the mineral content of soils from various districts in Finland showed that magnesium, calcium and potassium are much scarcer in the east, where mortality rates are highest, than in the southwest, where they are the lowest. The most pronounced difference, researchers reported, was in magnesium levels.

Another of their observations has been reported in a number of different studies. Samples of heart muscle taken from victims of heart attacks contain anywhere from 10 to 35 percent less magnesium than the hearts of those who died from other causes. Depleted magnesium levels in both humans and animals have also been associated with elevated blood pressure, that celebrated prelude to heart disease.

THE ANTISTRESS FACTOR

If magnesium deficiency really is one of the devils behind heart attacks, what factors affect the levels in our bodies, besides what we eat and what we drink? Well, it now appears that stress, that bugaboo of modern life, can have a marked effect on cellular magnesium levels. And of all the stresses the 20th century has accustomed us to, what could be more common, or more irritating, than noise?

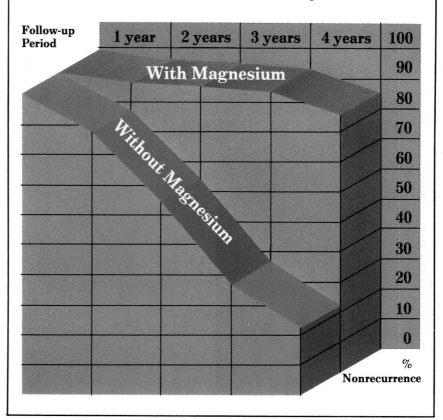

A Natural Cure for Kidney Stones

| Follow-up Period | 1 year | 2 years | 3 years | 4 years | 100 |

To test what effect prolonged noise stress might have on magnesium levels, German scientists at the federal health office in Berlin subjected five groups of rats to varying amounts of racket, up to levels that would drive any human batty: Several groups had to listen to tape-recorded traffic noise during 12 night hours for 12 weeks! Meanwhile, in their food and drinking water, the rats were fed levels of magnesium that were deficient in varying degrees.

At the end of the experiment, measurements showed that for all groups, "noise stress leads to a decrease of the cellular [magnesium] content and an increase of the [calcium] content." And the longer and louder the noise, the greater the decrease in magnesium levels. One group, subjected to traffic noise alternated with semiquiet periods, showed a 4 percent decrease in cellular magnesium. But the luckless bunch that was forced to listen to continuous noise, without any break at all, registered magnesium losses of 14 percent!

Similar results were found in people. After one working day with

Doctors in Sweden used magnesium to treat 56 people who chronically formed about 1 kidney stone a year. During the 4 years of the treatment, 86 percent of them were completely free from stones. Another group of 43 stone formers didn't get magnesium—and over 75 percent of them continued to get stones.

113

and one without loud traffic noise (85 decibels, or roughly the level of noise made by a kitchen garbage disposal unit), the scientists found "statistically significant alterations" in cellular magnesium levels.

On the other hand, studies have shown that even small increases in dietary magnesium seem to protect against noise-induced stress.

Is it possible that all kinds of stress drain the body's magnesium supply? Dr. Bella Altura suggests, for example, that the hard-charging, competitive behavior we call "Type A," known to be associated with an increased risk of heart attack, is really "a state of more-or-less constant self-induced stress"—and that what makes it so deadly is the self-induced depletion of magnesium.

MORE THAN JUST A HEART SAVER

Like most vital nutrients, magnesium performs more than one service to the body. In the same way that it protects against SDIHD, by blocking a calcium-induced contraction of the blood vessels, magnesium can also lower high blood pressure by dilating the blood vessels.

Many people would like to know how to prevent kidney stones, and magnesium might be the ticket there, also. Just as magnesium and calcium compete to maintain the relaxation/constriction balance of the heart, they apparently also compete for a place in the kidneys. Put simply, an optimum intake of magnesium can prevent a buildup of calcium deposits and the formation of calcium-based kidney stones, which account for two-thirds of all kidney stone cases in the United States.

In one study, 67 patients who had a tendency to form stones were given 500 milligrams of magnesium hydroxide daily and had a reduced rate of stone recurrence. (Five hundred milligrams of magnesium hydroxide equals approximately 200 milligrams of magnesium.) These findings suggest that magnesium lessens the chance of stone formation, the scientists who conducted the study reported during a conference of

the American College of Nutrition in St. Louis.

GETTING THE LEAD OUT

The problem of lead poisoning among inner-city or ghetto children might also be relieved by magnesium supplementation. Leonard F. Vitale, M.D., a pediatrician in the New York City area, and other researchers found that, in rats, "feeding magnesium leads to lower retention of and increased excretion of lead."

Magnesium won't remove lead already deposited in body tissue, Dr. Vitale says, but it might keep more from getting in.

Low levels of magnesium in the blood also may be an important risk factor in the development of a major complication of diabetes, Scandinavian researchers reported. The complication, called diabetic retinopathy, involves tiny hemorrhages in the retina of the eye that can lead to total blindness.

When a team of doctors in Denmark examined 71 insulin-treated diabetics who had had the eye disease for at least ten years, they found "a definite lowering" of blood magnesium levels, compared with 194 nondiabetics. And those patients with the most advanced and severe retinopathy had the lowest magnesium levels of all.

Last but not least, magnesium can rescue you from two commonplace but embarrassing conditions—bad breath and body odor. B. F. Hart, M.D., from Fort Lauderdale, Florida, claims that magnesium, when taken with zinc, PABA and vitamin B_6, can effectively control offensive body and breath odors.

WE ALL NEED MORE

Recommended allowances for magnesium range from 350 to 450 milligrams a day, but adult men in the United States ordinarily consume only about 75 percent of that. And a study of the diets of college students in Montreal revealed an average daily consumption of just 236 milligrams.

Why do so many people fall short? There are four basic reasons:

The Grain Drain

In one study, elderly folks ate iron-fortified grain products for several months. Yet their iron levels didn't go up 1 milligram.

Why? Because such foods are fortified with *ferric* iron (which is not absorbed) instead of *ferrous* iron (which occurs naturally in food and *is* absorbed).

The best way to put iron in your cereal bowl is to eat whole grains that contain iron naturally.

overprocessed food, soft water, synthetic fertilizers and destructive cooking practices.

"Traditionally, bulk cereals have been the most important source of dietary magnesium commonly available to man, but this cannot be said for contemporary overly refined food staples," the authors of a Canadian report said. For instance, whole wheat contains 1,502 ppm of magnesium, while white flour contains only 299 ppm.

In geographic areas where the drinking water is "soft" due to a lack of magnesium and other minerals, there is a higher rate of death from heart disease and a higher mortality rate in general. Towns in west Texas have the hardest drinking water and the lowest cardiovascular mortality rate in the United States. South Carolina, which has very soft water, also has the highest U.S. rate of cardiovascular death.

The use of synthetic fertilizers in agriculture since the turn of the century has had a depressing effect on the magnesium content of food. As crops draw minerals—including magnesium—from the soil, farmers often restore only the lost nitrogen, phosphorus and potassium.

Boiling vegetables can leach out their magnesium: one-half to three-fourths of the magnesium content of carrots, celery and parsnips can be found in their cooking water. Green vegetables generally contain adequate amounts of magnesium, but they should be steamed, baked or broiled.

To sum it all up, a magnesium-rich meal would contain one or more of these foods: whole grain bread, brown rice, spinach, corn, fresh fruit or a green vegetable, molasses or bran. A magnesium-poor meal could contain related foods, but ones denuded of nutrients: white bread or cake, white rice, boiled vegetables and canned fruit in heavy syrup.

ENERGIZE YOURSELF WITH IRON

It's a good bet that you may have a cast-iron skillet hanging on a hook or nestled in a cupboard in your kitchen. You've probably cooked with it

The Best Food Sources of Iron

Food	Portion	Iron (mg.)
Beef liver	3 oz.	7.5
Blackstrap molasses	1 tbsp.	3.2
Roast beef	3 oz.	3.1
Ground beef, lean	3 oz.	3.0
Lima beans, dried, cooked	½ cup	2.9
Sunflower seeds	¼ cup	2.6
Soybeans, dried, cooked	½ cup	2.5
Prunes	½ cup	2.2
Turkey, dark meat	3 oz.	2.0
Apricots, dried	¼ cup	1.8
Broccoli, raw	1 stalk	1.7
Spinach, raw, chopped	1 cup	1.7
Almonds, slivered	¼ cup	1.6
Peas, fresh, cooked	½ cup	1.5
Beet greens, cooked	½ cup	1.4
Brewer's yeast	1 tbsp.	1.4
Raisins	¼ cup	1.3
Kidney beans, dried, cooked	¼ cup	1.1
Turkey, white meat	3 oz.	1.1
Chicken, white meat	3 oz.	1.0
Endive or escarole, shredded	1 cup	1.0
Cod	3 oz.	0.9
Haddock	3 oz.	0.9

for years and bestowed upon it, omelet by omelet, a beautiful black patina. True, you can't see yourself in that skillet the way you can in one made of stainless steel. And, technologically, it's years behind space age nonstick cookware coatings. But the old skillet can give you something those other pans never will: iron. Very simply, when you cook in an iron pan, a little of the iron rubs off on your food.

And that's good, because a lot of us are just scraping by without as much iron as we need.

"People aren't dropping like flies from iron deficiency," one researcher says. "But if you're talking about optimum performance, no, we aren't getting as much iron as we should. With the amount of iron most of us are getting now, we're not going to feel as strong or as energetic or as

ARE YOU ANEMIC?

Iron deficiency anemia can sneak up and catch you napping—unless you know what to look for. Here are some clues:

- Apathy
- Brittle nails
- Depression
- Dizziness
- Fainting spells
- Fatigue
- Hair loss
- Headaches
- Heartburn
- Irritability
- Itching
- Pale lips
- Pale skin
- Poor appetite
- Rapid pulse
- Sore tongue
- Weak legs

alert as we could be."

Indeed, iron deficiency not only robs us of stamina but also weakens our resistance to infection, impairs our ability to learn and may promote stomach cancer and hair loss.

Doctors have known for centuries that a lack of iron in the diet or loss of iron through bleeding can cause weakness and fatigue. In ancient times, physicians prescribed sweet wine laced with iron filings to revive wounded warriors. In recent times, researchers have taken field trips to tea plantations in Sri Lanka (Ceylon) and to garment factories in the Philippines to discover whether undernourished workers become significantly more productive after receiving iron supplements. In one such experiment on a tea plantation in Sri Lanka, scientists determined that work productivity *did* improve when people were given daily iron supplements. The degree of improvement in work output seemed to be greater in those workers whose iron levels were lowest before the experiment.

The researchers also measured the level of physical activity of anemic plantation workers in their everyday environment before and after iron supplementation. They reported that, after three weeks, the activity levels "were significantly greater in the iron-treated than in matched placebo-treated subjects." Their data also provided "strong evidence for the clinical impression that people with iron deficiency anemia suffer from tiredness and weakness."

Why does iron affect physical performance? Partly because of a specific reddish-brown, iron-containing protein in the blood called hemoglobin. As hemoglobin passes through the blood vessels of the lungs, it grabs hold of oxygen molecules and carries them to the tissues, where each cell uses it to produce energy. Just as a candle will go out if you cover it with a jar, the microscopic fire in each cell will go out if you deprive it of oxygen. Without iron, the body can't produce hemoglobin, and without hemoglobin, only a trace of oxygen will reach the cells. The condition that results from hemoglobin-poor blood is called anemia.

DIRECT ACTION ON MUSCLES

Yet iron's effect on energy may not be limited to perking up tired blood; the muscles themselves may need adequate iron to function properly.

That discovery came from Sweden in the course of a study of the effects of iron supplementation on the work capacity of healthy men and women between the ages of 58 and 71. Half were given iron supplements twice daily for a period of three months, and half were given a placebo. Throughout the three months, their capacity for work was measured using an exercise bicycle, and the performance of the two groups was compared.

While the average work performance improved in both groups, the improvement was about *four times greater* in the group taking iron. But researcher Per Ericsson reported that "In spite of the fact that there was a significant increase in physical work capacity in the iron-supplemented group, no correlations were found between the increase in physical work capacity and the initial values or changes of other measures of the state of iron nutrition."

(As we said before, the usual measures of iron nutrition are those which are connected with the role it plays in the formation of red blood cells. The most common of these is the measurement of the amount of hemoglobin in the blood.)

The Swedish researchers found that iron supplementation increased the ability to perform physical work even in people who initially showed no signs that they needed more iron. More important, the iron supplementation caused no significant changes in levels of hemoglobin. People with relatively low hemoglobin levels *did not* develop higher levels after taking iron. The improvement in physical performance seemed to have nothing to do with what was happening in the blood.

It's this possibility that a team of researchers at the University of Washington has explored. They used a special transfusion procedure with rats to test the effects of iron supplementation independent of the levels of hemoglobin in the blood.

They trained the rats to use a small animal treadmill, then surgically inserted a catheter through which they transfused blood to maintain a uniform level of hemoglobin.

"At a hemoglobin compatible with normal work performance," one of the investigators, Clement A. Finch, M.D., reported, "iron-deficient animals showed a marked impairment of running ability as compared to control animals. Iron therapy corrected the disability within four days." Even with the same levels of hemoglobin, animals that were not getting enough iron in their diets were unable to perform as well as rats receiving sufficient iron. The effects of iron on physical performance, Dr. Finch concluded, are as much the result of direct action on the *muscles* as they are the result of the action of iron-generated hemoglobin. "It was evident," he wrote, "that muscle dysfunction exists in iron deficiency of sufficient severity but is ordinarily hidden by anemia."

THE BRAIN NEEDS IRON

Iron deficiency can also lead to impaired memory. One study has shown that children with even a mild iron shortage have poorer memory and learn less quickly than kids with adequate iron.

"One of the behavioral consequences of iron deficiency is an impairment of mental function," says Thomas F. Massaro, Ph.D., of Pennsylvania State University. "This has been demonstrated both in laboratory animals and in children. Children with a subclinical iron deficiency *can* learn—they won't be retarded— but the deficiency will interfere with *what* they learn."

For instance, if you send children with plenty of hemoglobin coursing through their veins into a room and later ask them to report what they saw there, they will remember and name clocks and lamps and rugs and books and many other things, Dr. Massaro says. But an iron-deficient child might remember far fewer objects in the room. Iron deficiency creates a kind of intellectual tunnel vision. Fortunately, a child's iron-related learning

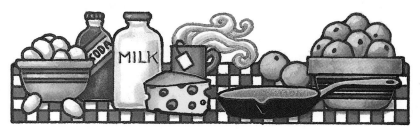

Iron Enemies—Iron Friends

How well your body uses the iron in the foods you eat depends on what else is on the menu. Some foods increase the amount of iron your body absorbs, while others make the mineral unavailable.

Do you eat a lot of ice cream, candy bars and baked goods or drink a lot of beer or soft drinks? Phosphates in those foods block iron absorption.

In fact, the more canned or processed the food you eat, the more you consume EDTA, another additive that tangles up dietary iron.

Dairy products are wonderful sources of calcium, but eating too much cheese and yogurt or drinking too much milk interferes with the uptake of iron. Eggs, too, contain an anti-iron factor that binds it up not only in eggs but also in foods eaten with eggs—like toast. And the tannic acid in tea is a very powerful blocker of iron, too.

On the plus side are a host of foods that enhance iron absorption. At the top of the list is meat. Beef, poultry, fish, lamb, veal and game all multiply iron absorption fourfold. These meats help your body use nonheme iron, a form of the mineral that's found in *many* foods but isn't easy to absorb.

Citrus fruits, vegetables like cabbage, peppers, tomatoes and broccoli, plus cantaloupe and strawberries *all* encourage the uptake of nonheme iron because they all contain ample vitamin C, which also helps us to better utilize the nonheme form.

Vegetables and citrus fruits also contain folate, a B vitamin that iron needs to work well. Liver, beans and seafood, too, are high in folate.

Cooking food in an iron pot also can help boost iron intake by 3 or 4 times, thanks to iron contributed as the food simmers.

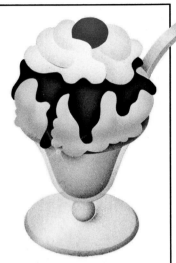

Keep Your Sweet Tooth Sharp

Getting all the zinc you need might be one way to cut down on sugar. In one study, people who received zinc supplements experienced a dramatic improvement in their ability to taste sweetness. These were ordinary, healthy people with no outward signs of zinc deficiency. That means zinc can help you become more sensitive to sweetness, and thus require less sugar to achieve the same taste.

disabilities can be corrected with about four months of iron supplementation.

A DIAGNOSIS THAT'S OFTEN MISSED

Even though anemia causes a host of problems, doctors rarely hit the nail on the head when it comes to diagnosing an iron deficiency.

They'll nod knowledgeably that women—especially menstruating women—face a greater risk of depleting their iron stores than men. They readily admit that an iron deficiency is sometimes the cause of vague and misleading symptoms. And they're the first to recognize anemia as the last straw in iron deficiency.

Yet how many young women suffering from fatigue, irritability, dizziness or headaches (all symptoms of iron deficiency) drag themselves to their doctors for assistance and slouch away with little more than an "it's-all-in-your-head" diagnosis and a catchall prescription for tranquilizers?

We'd venture to say, quite a few. Not that headaches or irritability can't be brought on by a bout with nervous tension. But, according to statistics from the National Institute on Drug Abuse, physicians are twice as eager to lay the blame on nerves when it involves a female patient— even though one specialist points out that one-third to one-half of apparently healthy young women are in fact iron depleted.

Although that worn-out, rundown feeling is the most common symptom of an iron deficiency, it's by no means the only one. And it's not the first one doctors have mistaken for an emotional disturbance.

Why does iron deficiency produce such a curious array of symptoms? And why are these symptoms frequently overlooked as a warning signal?

"The symptoms of an iron deficiency are individualized and you don't have to be at the point of severe anemia to feel the effects," says James Cook, M.D., professor of medicine and director of hematology at the University of Kansas Medical Center. "I've seen patients with marked anemia who didn't seem to have *any* symptoms, and others with only slightly depressed iron levels who came to my office complaining of any number of related problems."

Many times it's not easy to diagnose an iron deficiency. "I know of cases where people suffering from appreciable fatigue responded to iron therapy even though initial blood tests did not show an abnormally low hemoglobin level," says Dr. Cook. "This is not, of course, to say that some people feign improvement. It's just that what is considered normal for one person may represent an iron deficiency in another. The key is individualized hemoglobin levels."

But how much iron does the body need to keep hemoglobin levels up to par?

Well, according to Dr. Cook, that depends on many varying factors. For example, if you're an average American male, you're probably on pretty solid ground. The iron in your daily diet more than compensates for the 1 milligram of iron that is lost daily via the skin and the urinary and gastrointestinal tracts, he says.

But if you've an average American female, your health could be balancing on a precarious tightrope. Data from a nationwide survey by the U.S. Department of Health and Human Services revealed that 95 percent of American women aged 18 to 44 are not getting enough iron— only a little more than half of the Recommended Dietary Allowance set at 18 milligrams for menstruating women.

Why?

To begin with, a woman generally eats less than a man—which means less iron. And if she's trimming her waistline by cutting down on iron-rich foods like meat and cereal and substituting such poor iron sources as skim milk, yogurt and cottage cheese, then her iron intake is sure to fall short.

But it's not bad enough that she's getting less iron from her diet than a man. Her body requires more—almost twice as much to make up for monthly losses during normal menstruation.

And that doesn't take into account special circumstances, like the excessive blood loss of menorrhagia (heavy or prolonged menstrual bleeding) caused by physiological problems or the use of certain intrauterine devices for contraception. Or the regular use of aspirin, which tends to cause irritation and bleeding of the stomach lining. Or the drain of maternal nutrient stores during pregnancy. In addition, there are several stages of life when iron requirements increase.

The growth spurt between infancy and adolescence is one. In fact, according to Mississippi State University home economists Catherine C. Johnson and Mary F. Futrell, Ph.D., iron deficiency anemia is "the most prevalent nutritional disorder among children in the United States."

Anemia knows no generation gap, either. Our senior citizens are at risk as well. Of a group of 484 elderly persons in a nursing home and hospital, 151 (31 percent) had anemia or were receiving therapy for anemia—of which iron deficiency anemia was the most common type—according to two Toronto investigators. Much of the iron problem in general is the result of limited absorption of the mineral. People usually absorb only 5 to 10 percent of the iron they eat in food, but the absorption of iron is greatly influenced by the foods it is eaten with. Dr. Cook has done extensive work on the absorption of iron, and believes the kind of food you eat with your iron can make the difference between adequate intake of the nutrient and iron deficiency. Vitamin C, for instance, can increase absorption fourfold.

It's a good thing to have tricks like this up your sleeve. You've got to stay on your toes when you're dealing with iron deficiency, even if the problem seems kind of old hat. There's no room for complacency, or a false sense of security. (For more information on iron absorption, see the box on page 117.)

THINK ZINC

Two decades ago, few people— including doctors and nutritionists— were even aware of zinc and its role in our diet.

The Best Food Sources of Zinc

Food	Portion	Zinc (mg.)
Chicken heart	3 oz.	6.3
Beef, lean	3 oz.	5.3
Calves' liver	3 oz.	5.2
Beef liver	3 oz.	4.4
Lamb, lean	3 oz.	4.3
Ground beef, lean	3 oz.	3.8
Chicken liver	3 oz.	3.7
Turkey, dark meat	3 oz.	3.5
Pumpkin seeds	¼ cup	2.6
Chicken, dark meat	3 oz.	2.4
Swiss cheese	2 oz.	2.2
Sunflower seeds	¼ cup	2.0
Brazil nuts	¼ cup	1.8
Cheddar cheese	2 oz.	1.8
Turkey, white meat	3 oz.	1.8
Black-eyed peas, dried, cooked	½ cup	1.5
Cashews	¼ cup	1.5
Oats, rolled	½ cup	1.4
Soybeans, dried, cooked	½ cup	1.3
Peanuts, roasted	¼ cup	1.2
Chicken, white meat	3 oz.	1.1
Peas, dried, cooked	½ cup	1.1
Chick-peas, dried, cooked	½ cup	1.0
Lentils, dried, cooked	½ cup	1.0

Today we know that no one can hope to be healthy without it. Zinc helps conditions as varied as night vision, prostate function, the senses of taste and smell and even wound healing (zinc's the stuff in calamine lotion that soothes your poison ivy rash). It appears to reduce inflammation, clear up acne and tone down body odor. It's important to proper growth and sexual maturity, crucial to the body's protein-manufacturing factories and is vital to the functioning of some 90 enzymes, those chemical traffic cops that help regulate dozens of bodily processes every day. Our roundup of zinc benefits begins defensively—with the immune system.

Infection and Immunity. A report in the *American Journal of Clinical Nutrition* confirms previous evidence that zinc can boost the body's immune response. A 17-year-old boy hospitalized for a severe head injury had developed a zinc deficiency in the course of being tube-fed. Tests indicated that the lymphocyte cells, key components of the immune system which protect against disease-carrying organisms, were not functioning normally. Zinc supplementation was begun at the rate of approximately 22 milligrams per day, and within three weeks lymphocyte response bounced back to normal.

As an additional bonus, a facial inflammation and an ulceration on the youth's ankle also cleared up promptly.

Zinc's role in the fight against infection is of special interest to older people. Aging, unfortunately, tends to increase your risk of "immunologic deficiency"—a rather dull way of saying you're outgunned in a shoot-out with disease. Because of this, a group of Belgian researchers tested the effect of oral zinc supplements on 15 patients over 70 years old, to see if zinc would improve their ability to fight off infection.

For a month, the 15 elderly people were given 220 milligrams of zinc sulfate (equivalent to 50 milligrams of elemental zinc) twice a day. This dosage, the doctors reported, was "well tolerated," though 5 patients experienced bouts of nausea and mild diarrhea. Three tests of the immune system's strength were used to compare the zinc group with 15 untreated controls: total number of circulating T-lymphocytes; skin reaction to a specific invader; and production of antibodies (or antigen-specific attackers) in response to tetanus vaccine.

The zinc group, the researchers found, showed a "significant improvement" in all three areas. "The data suggest," they concluded, "that the addition of zinc to the diet of old persons could be an effective and simple way to improve their immune function."

Wound Healing. Chronic leg ulcerations and other stubborn, slow-to-heal wounds have been helped dramatically when extra zinc was added to the diet. "If one considers that wound healing is a process in which active cell growth and protein synthesis are occurring, it is not surprising that a deficiency of a nutrient essential for normal growth would result in impaired wound healing," says Philip A. Walravens, M.D., of the University of Colorado Medical Center in Denver.

Unfortunately, the very people who need zinc most are likely to be the most deficient. After burns and other serious injuries, large amounts of zinc are excreted in the urine. And hospital patients frequently suffer from zinc deficiency before and after surgery.

Pollution. Zinc can also prevent the toxic effects of cadmium, a heavy metal that pollutes our air, water and food and accumulates in the body. In one study, scientists fed young quail a diet containing cadmium. When zinc was added to the diet, the level of cadmium in the tissues dropped.

"Zinc is an important element in preventing the accretion [accumulation] of low levels of cadmium similar to those present in the diet of man," wrote the scientists in the journal *Federation Proceedings.*

Fertility and Sexual Potency. Zinc has been used successfully to improve fertility. Ali A. Abbasi, M.D., an endocrinologist formerly at the Allen Park Veterans' Administration Hospital in Michigan and now in private practice, showed that even a mild zinc deficiency caused sperm counts to drop below the point of technical sterility. Supplemental zinc, however, returned sperm counts to normal.

Low semen zinc levels have also been associated with poor sperm motility. But Joel L. Marmar, M.D., a Cherry Hill, New Jersey, urologist, reported boosting the sperm motility index (percent and quality of sperm that move) an average of 33 percent by giving zinc sulfate to men with low semen zinc levels.

Kidney patients who undergo long-term treatment on an artificial kidney machine often complain of impotence and diminished sex drive. At the same time, zinc levels in their blood decline. So a team of researchers at the Veterans' Administration Hospital and Georgetown University School of Medicine in Washington, D.C., decided to add supplemental zinc via the kidney machine's dialysis bath.

Results were gratifying. Three of the four men receiving zinc reported a striking improvement in potency two weeks after the treatment began. The fourth patient improved after four weeks.

Sense of Taste. Zinc plays an important role in taste perception. Studies have shown that people who have difficulty tasting their food (hypogeusia is the technical term) often have reduced levels of zinc in their blood and saliva. That can lead to a vicious cycle, since loss of taste reduces appetite and thus lessens the likelihood of correcting the zinc deficiency through food intake alone. But when supplemental zinc is provided, full taste sensation and appetite can sometimes be restored within a month.

Night Vision. One common eye disorder that can be caused by zinc deficiency is night blindness, the inability of the eyes to adapt to darkness. In a study of six men with night blindness, all regained normal vision after taking zinc supplements for two weeks. Doctors believe that zinc corrects night vision by converting vitamin A to its active form, retinaldehyde, in the retina.

Rheumatoid Arthritis. Although a truly effective cure for this crippling disease continues to elude medical science, there is at least preliminary evidence that some people may be helped by zinc. In a study reported by Peter A. Simkin, M.D., of the University of Washington's division of rheumatology, a group of patients receiving supplemental zinc noted less joint swelling, reduced morning stiffness and improved walking speed compared with others not taking zinc. Those beneficial changes occurred within the first 12 weeks of treatment. During the following 12 weeks, there was also "an impressive reduction in joint tenderness."

Dr. Simkin hypothesizes that the extra zinc may somehow produce

Zinc Protects the Prostate

The prostate gland produces launching fluid for sperm cells. If the gland swells, it pinches off the urethra, increasing the urge to urinate and causing burning pain, false starts, dribbling and inability to void. The same difficulties arise when the prostate is infected and inflamed (prostatitis).

Prostate woes are no small matter—they plague more than 60 percent of all men over age 60.

Taking zinc may end all that misery, though. Irving M. Bush, M.D., of Chicago's Cook County Hospital, has had good results treating men with enlarged prostate (benign prostate hypertrophy) with 34 milligrams of zinc a day for 2 months. All 19 men studied experienced easing of symptoms, and swelling subsided in all but 5 men.

Zinc also has antibacterial properties that may protect against prostate infections. Warren Heston, Ph.D., research assistant professor of urology at the Washington University School of Medicine in St. Louis, reported that he and his colleagues found that the prostatic fluid of men with prostatitis had only about one-tenth as much zinc as fluid of men free of prostate trouble.

Dr. Heston says that men with prostatitis seem to have a "turned off" prostate, and that zinc may be the mechanism that turns it back on.

an anti-inflammatory effect in the synovial membrane around joints.

BRIGHTEN YOUR HEALTH WITH CHROMIUM

You need so little chromium that it's measured in micrograms. Do you know how tiny that is? Imagine this. You conscientiously consume all the chromium your body requires every day—at the most, 200 micrograms. Now, if you added all those daily chromium quantities together it would take an incredible *5,000* days (more than 13 years) before they totaled just one single gram—and *that* would fit on the tip of your finger with room to spare!

Our chromium requirements may be small, but as a protector against cardiovascular disease and diabetes, chromium's impact is likely to be quite significant. In fact, atherosclerosis is the most common cause of death among diabetics.

"It seems that insulin problems are what link these two deadly diseases together," says Richard A. Anderson, Ph.D., of the USDA's Human Nutrition Research Center, Beltsville, Maryland.

"Insulin is required to remove glucose from the blood. When sugar levels in the blood are high, the pancreas dispatches insulin, which stimulates the cells to take up the glucose and burn it for energy. Chromium makes insulin more efficient at this task, so you need less to accomplish the job," explains Dr. Anderson. "And that's beneficial, because high insulin levels in the blood are thought to be associated with hardening of the arteries."

"The chromium/insulin/atherosclerosis connection is quite significant," adds Howard A. I. Newman, Ph.D., professor of pathology at Ohio State University College of Medicine. "Samples of human aortas from areas of the world where atherosclerosis is mild or virtually absent contain more chromium than do aortas from [people in] areas where the disease is more prevalent." And when chromium concentrations were measured in the aortas of accident victims, they were found to be significantly greater than in aortas of people who died from atherosclerotic heart disease (also known as coronary artery disease).

Rebecca Riales, Ph.D., a nutritionist from Parkersburg, West Virginia, tested the effect of chromium supplementation on glucose tolerance, insulin and serum lipids, including HDL cholesterol (the good kind).

The experiment lasted 12 weeks and during that time, the 23 adult men (aged 31 to 60) in the study were given either 200 micrograms of chromium or a placebo for five days each week. By the end of the experiment there was a significant increase in HDL cholesterol in the chromium group. What's more, there was also a decrease in body weight and a trend toward decreased triglycerides and insulin levels. The placebo group showed none of those positive effects.

As for glucose tolerance (the ability of the body to clear glucose from the bloodstream), that improved somewhat in the chromium-supplemented group, too.

"It all fits together," Dr. Riales says. "And while it's still only theory, the evidence gets stronger every day. Chromium is part of a substance called glucose tolerance factor (GTF). Here it acts sort of like a gasket

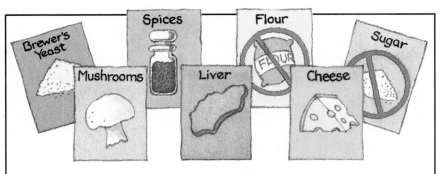

Conserve Your Chromium

Even if you're eating plenty of high-chromium foods like brewer's yeast, liver, cheese, chili peppers, mushrooms and potatoes, you still may be losing out on the mineral if you eat refined carbohydrates or drink too much milk—or both.

Loading up on white flour and white sugar steals chromium by stepping up insulin production, which in turn flushes out chromium. To protect the chromium you've got, stay away from sugary desserts, white flour products, syrups and candy.

Like iron, chromium is bound up into undigestible forms when it meets up with the phosphates in milk—and then it passes right through you, unused. So to protect the chromium you do get, go easy on the milk when you're feasting on chromium-rich foods.

between insulin and its receptor sites on cell membranes. So if there's a mild chromium deficiency, then insulin can't bind as well to its receptors and sugar can't be cleared as well from the blood.

"But," she continues, "there's also an enzyme attached to vessel walls that clears fat from the bloodstream. That enzyme requires insulin for its activation. So if insulin is not working up to par (due to lack of chromium) then these blood fats do not get cleared as well.

"Our findings support the hypothesis that chromium deficiency could be one factor in the genesis of decreased HDL cholesterol, hyperinsulinemia [elevated blood insulin levels] and insulin resistance, and through these changes, of atherosclerosis," Dr. Riales wrote in the *American Journal of Clinical Nutrition.*

So how do we know who is chromium deficient? Victoria J. K. Liu, Ph.D., of Purdue University, found that people who have high insulin levels are much more likely to have low chromium levels.

This has some important implications for individuals in the early stages of maturity-onset diabetes. These people actually have very high insulin levels. But their insulin is inefficient and can't do the work it's supposed to do. When they are given chromium, both their sugar and insulin levels go down.

"Our hypothesis is that certain people with normal glucose tolerance may have a progressive elevation of serum levels and decrease of chromium response," says Dr. Liu. "When the condition advances to a certain point, an abnormal glucose tolerance may come into sight, and the abnormality can be reversed in some cases with chromium supplementation."

Research has shown that chromium may be linked with a few other, less life-threatening problems as well—such as wound healing. Dr. Liu conducted a study to compare the healing time between rats fed a low-chromium diet and those fed a high-chromium diet. Fifteen days following minor surgery, wound healing was significantly less advanced in the low-chromium group and they had also gained significantly less weight per unit of food eaten.

The Best Food Sources of Chromium*

Excellent	Brewer's yeast	Calves' liver
Good	Potatoes with skin Beef Fresh vegetables	Whole grain bread Cheese Chicken legs
Fair	Fresh fruit Chicken breast	Fish and seafood

*NOTE: Nutritional science has yet to quantify the exact amount of chromium in foods; that's why this food source table is a little different from the others.

Dr. Anderson of the USDA has done some additional chromium research, too. His study took a look at the effects of a dietary chromium deficiency on the sperm count and fertility of rats. By the age of eight months, the rats raised on a low-chromium diet had only half as much sperm as animals raised on a chromium-supplemented diet. Not only that, the frequency of conception was less than that of the high-chromium group.

As for the effect on people, Dr. Anderson says, "I wouldn't be surprised at all if a chromium deficiency affects male sperm counts and fertility in the same way it affects rats."

Even though a tiny amount of chromium is needed for optimum health—about 50 to 200 micrograms per day—it's not that simple to obtain in the diet.

"About one-third of the population gets less than that amount," says Dr. Anderson. "What's more, eating too much sugar and other simple carbohydrates over a long period of time can stimulate chromium losses. We are concerned that the high levels of sugar in our American diet, along with the increased consumption of highly processed foods that are usually low in chromium, may be leading to serious dietary chromium deficiencies."

SELENIUM: PROMISING WEAPON AGAINST CANCER

All of us, every day, absorb small amounts of carcinogens—substances that can cause cancer. Lead from auto exhaust, PCBs in the food chain, even by-products of our own digestion—all can do us harm. They penetrate our cells and attack the cell nuclei, promoting cancer by scrambling the genetic code that programs us for health.

We can't stop that steady rain of pollution, but we can put up an umbrella. There's new evidence that the trace element selenium protects cell membranes, cell nuclei and chromosomes from damage.

There are several theories about what selenium does, on the cellular level, to prevent cancer. John A. Milner, Ph.D., of the University of Illinois, Urbana-Champaign, speculates that selenium's effect on rapidly dividing cells might explain why his laboratory mice didn't get cancer when they received selenium supplements.

Dr. Milner transplanted cancer cells into healthy mice and then injected some of them with selenium salts. After six weeks, all of the unsupplemented mice were bloated with tumors and were double their original weight, but the supplemented mice were trim, healthy and tumor free. Selenium continued to protect the mice for three weeks after supplementation stopped. "Complete inhibition of tumor development was observed for all selenium compounds administered at a dose of 2 micrograms per gram of body weight," wrote Dr. Milner in *Science*.

Dr. Milner says that his study results might have "profound implications" for cancer prevention. He suspects that selenium somehow slows the growth of cancer cells without affecting healthy cells.

The possibility that selenium slows down cell division also interests Gerhard Schrauzer, Ph.D., a chemistry professor at the University of California's Revelle College and perhaps that nation's leading selenium researcher. He believes selenium prevents cancer partly by delaying cell division long enough for a carcinogen-damaged cell to repair its chromosomes.

Dr. Schrauzer estimates that among people who don't smoke or otherwise expose themselves to large doses of carcinogens, an adequate supply of selenium provides effective resistance to cancers of the intestine, rectum, breast, ovary, prostate, lung, pancreas, skin, kidney and bladder, as well as to certain types of leukemia. Selenium does this, he says, not only by retarding cell division, but also by promoting the production of glutathione peroxidase (GSH-px), an enzyme that turns peroxides (reactive particles that can destroy a cell) into harmless water. It may also aid in the production of interferon, the body's natural antiviral and anticancer drug.

NEW HOPE FOR BREAST CANCER

Selenium may be a special blessing to women with breast cancer. It seems as if selenium can counteract some of the cancer-causing effects of fat, and one thing researchers agree on is that high-fat diets provide a breeding ground for breast tumors.

Animals in a study were divided into two groups. Those in the high-fat group were placed on diets consisting of 25 percent fat; those in the low-fat group were fed a modest 5 percent fat. The average American diet, by the way, should fall somewhere between 25 and 30 percent—but it actually contains a whopping 42 percent fat.

All the animals received selenium supplements, in amounts ranging from 5 to 25 times their daily requirement. They were also given a chemical that would induce breast tumor development.

Astoundingly, animals in the high-fat group that received 25 times their daily requirement of selenium experienced fewer tumors than those in the low-fat group that received only 5 times the daily requirement. The researchers also noted that tumors took longer to develop in the animals given the most selenium. "In conclusion," they wrote in *Cancer Research*, "high dietary selenium levels are able to protect against mammary tumorigenesis, but rats on a high-fat diet still develop more tumors than those on a low-fat diet at comparable selenium supplementation."

The earlier selenium supplementation begins, the better, Dr. Schrauzer believes. "Dietary selenium prevents and retards tumor development," he reports, "only as long as it is supplied in adequate amounts. . . . Maximum protection is achieved if supplementation is introduced early and maintained over the entire life span of the animals. However, a 'late' protective effect of selenium is still apparent."

Most significantly, if selenium can prevent breast tumors in mice, Dr. Schrauzer says, it may prevent them in humans. In partial confirmation of that theory, researchers elsewhere have found that breast cancer patients have "significantly" less selenium in their blood than do healthy women.

Selenium's broadest role may lie in protecting our cells from the low-level but constant barrage of carcinogens hidden in our air, food and water. In this regard, Dr. Schrauzer calls selenium an "environmental protecting agent."

That view is shared by researchers at the University of Southern California's School of Pharmacy. In experiments with rats, they found that selenium supplementation had a "significant protective effect" against low doses of a chemical carcinogen.

Selenium has two vitamin "helpers"—A and E. Together, selenium and vitamin A have a stronger effect against breast tumors than either alone. And, interestingly, vitamin E has a "sparing effect" on selenium. If a person's vitamin E supply is high, he'll need less selenium. Raymond Shamberger, Ph.D., of the Cleveland Clinic Foundation, explains that vitamin E may "stabilize selenium, keeping it in a form that the body can use more easily."

So if you are taking selenium to guard against breast cancer, you would be wise to take vitamins A and E as well.

Selenium appears to be in short supply in our diet, because of soil deficiencies and poor personal food choices. But because it is required only in trace amounts (*too much* could actually be harmful), recommended supplementation levels are

Selenium and Breast Cancer: A Link?

States with Highest Incidence of Breast Cancer

States with Lowest Levels of Selenium in Soil

quite modest. Dr. Schrauzer estimates that dietary selenium intake should be doubled. This could be done by increasing consumption of selenium-rich foods such as seafood, whole grain cereal and bread products and organ meats like kidney and liver. Yeast supplements specially cultured to contain higher amounts of biologically active selenium are also available.

The raised states in the bottom map have *low* levels of selenium. The raised states in the top map have *high* levels of breast cancer. As you can see, they're almost a perfect match, a fact that's led many scientists to say low selenium is probably a risk factor in the disease.

9

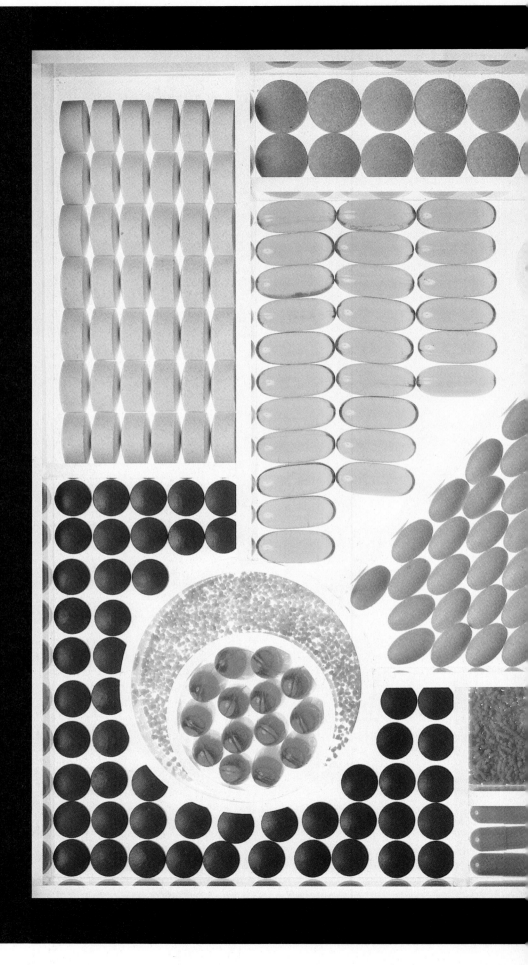

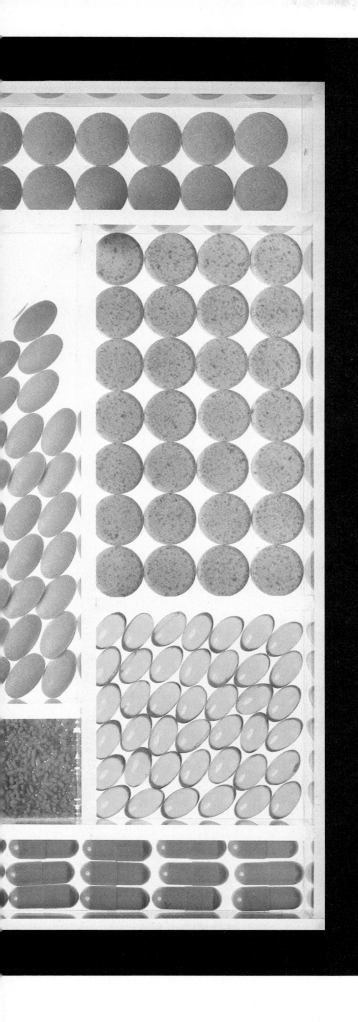

The Special Supplements

Our 4-star rating system is your guide to these unique health products.

One of them is made up of friendly bacteria, tiny organisms that live in your intestines and help regulate digestion. Another is a cousin to the charcoal bricks you use in your barbecue. A third is squeezed from the livers of fish. Others come from giant weeds beneath the sea, or the root of an herb that can sell for hundreds of dollars, or the food that worker bees gather to feed the young in a hive.

But as exotic and varied as these substances are, they all have one thing in common: They're not vitamins or minerals, yet you can find them among the nutritional supplements in a typical health food store. Why are they there?

Because people believe that they work.

But belief is one thing, fact another. There are plenty of doctors who say the public is being gulled by ridiculous claims into paying top dollar for worthless supplements. In some cases, that's true, and we've weeded those supplements out of this chapter. But in other cases, the supplements *are* worthwhile. *How* worthwhile is the real question.

To answer it, we've devised a rating system that uses four stars. *One star* means the supplement might do you some good; there's a little scientific evidence, but nothing to write home about. *Two stars* mean that the scientific proof that supports the product's usefulness is somewhat stronger, but the verdict is not unanimous. *Three stars* are a different ballgame, meaning that studies have consistently proven the therapeutic power of the substance, and many people may benefit from taking it. *Four stars* indicate both the strongest positive evidence and the greatest likelihood of benefit.

Acidophilus ★★★

Acidophilus is actually a strain of bacteria—a beneficial one that naturally inhabits the stomach and bowel—but a "germ" nonetheless. Despite its lineage, it can be helpful in a number of health situations—most of them involving digestion and bowel function—when used regularly and in any one of its variety of forms. Acidophilus bacteria can be taken either in fermented milk products like yogurt and sweet acidophilus milk or as a concentrated supplement.

In its simplest form of direct health action, these bacteria—whether taken by themselves or in a milk product—work on the milk protein casein, making it easier to digest. And for people with an intolerance to milk sugar (lactose), those friendly bacteria make it possible to eat yogurt and drink sweet acidophilus milk because the bacteria digest the lactose for them.

Acidophilus bacteria also help maintain normal bowel function even when there's no digestion to be done. A team of researchers at the University of Nebraska's department of food science and technology has discovered a natural antibiotic activity in some strains of *Lactobacillus acidophilus*. This natural antibiotic, which they refer to as "acidophilin," inhibited 27 different types of bacteria, including strep, staph and salmonella.

The presence of these infection fighters in the intestine is important in another way, too. When they're on guard they can also fight diarrhea, whether it arises from an adverse food reaction or the use of antibiotic drugs. As we heard one nutrition-oriented doctor tell a patient with both a bladder infection and diarrhea, "Acidophilus bacteria are vital to restoring your internal body ecology to normal. When you take antibiotics, they kill the germs you don't want, in your case the infectious ones in your bladder. But they also kill many perfectly normal, indispensable bacteria that live in your intestines. These friendly bacteria help digest food, produce essential vitamins and help keep bowel function normal. If they're not replaced, symptoms such as yours are frequent, particularly with repeated courses of antibiotics.

"But whether you have symptoms or not, anytime you take antibiotics for any reason they should always be followed by an acidophilus chaser. Acidophilus won't interfere with your antibiotics, and it helps keep your internal body ecology normal." The doctor went on to advise this particular patient to take a tablespoon of liquid acidophilus or three or four capsules twice daily for at least two to three weeks because she'd been having her problem for some time.

Another doctor, writing to the medical journal *Lancet,* reported that antibiotic therapy also destroys the protective acidophilus in the vagina, and that women with vaginal infections should take the bacteria. "I have used it for this purpose for over 30 years," he wrote, and it has proved to be "very effective." He also described an added benefit: "In three such women who also had a history of lifelong eczema, giving the lactobacillus [acidophilus] caused the skin to clear completely."

One final annoyance that acidophilus has been known to banish is the cold sore. The virus causing cold sores (herpes simplex) is quickly crowded out by the friendly bacteria.

Acidophilus, the friendly type of bacteria that aids digestion, doesn't come only in supplement form. You also can get it from yogurt (some brands don't have it, so check the ingredients). Or you could drink sweet acidophilus milk, formulated so it does not have the acidophilus tang.

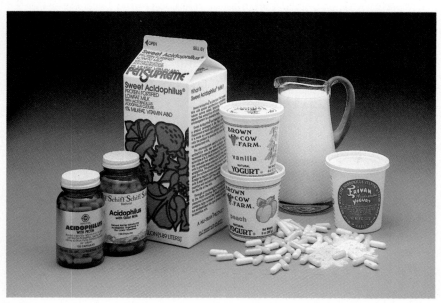

128

Alfalfa ★★

Wouldn't it be great to have a treatment for the cholesterol problem that would work even if we ate considerably more fat than was good for us? Well, alfalfa at least *tries.* New animal research shows that when the diet is supplemented with generous amounts of alfalfa, cholesterol deposits are "scrubbed out" of the arteries even when cholesterol is being ingested in amounts ordinarily sufficient to *cause* fatty deposits.

This research was carried out on a large group of monkeys at the Oregon Regional Primate Research Center in Beaverton, Oregon, and the Cleveland Clinic Foundation in Cleveland, Ohio, by a team of scientists supervised by M. R. Malinow, M.D. In the first stage of the experiment, the monkeys were given a good dose of atherosclerosis by feeding them lots of cholesterol.

Following that, the animals were divided into diet groups: straight commercial monkey chow; a semi-purified diet containing cholesterol; and the same cholesterol diet plus 50 percent alfalfa meal.

As might be expected, the animals that received no cholesterol and simply ate the commercial chow had very few signs of atherosclerosis, while the group fed cholesterol without anything protective in the diet developed the worst damage. But the really interesting find was that the animals receiving cholesterol plus alfalfa had, at autopsy, arteries as "clean" as those of the monkeys that were fed only monkey chow and no cholesterol at all!

The amount of cholesterol fed to these animals was "comparable to the habitual diet of man in the U.S.," the researchers pointed out. However, we have to stress that alfalfa in these experiments was given as 50 percent of the diet, an amount greater than any man, we think, would or could eat as part of his daily fare. (In fact, it would probably be poisonous.) So at least two questions remain. The first is whether alfalfa has the same effect on humans that it does on monkeys. No one knows, of course. The second question is proba-

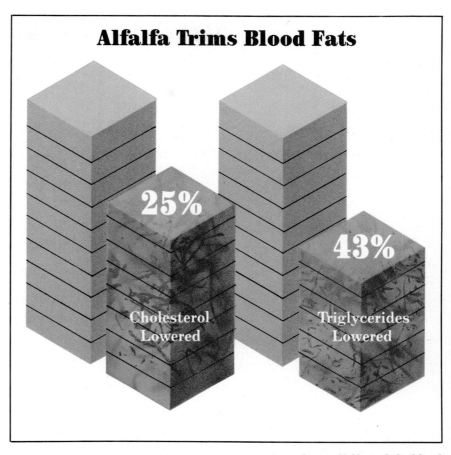

Alfalfa Trims Blood Fats

25% Cholesterol Lowered

43% Triglycerides Lowered

bly more critical, and that is *how much* alfalfa a person would have to eat in order to obtain some meaningful benefit from this plant. Again, we can only guess.

Scientists studying alfalfa—and there are a number of them besides the investigators who carried out this particular study—are probably more interested in yet another question: What exact part of the alfalfa plant, or what chemical naturally occurring in alfalfa, is responsible for its anticholesterol action? One thing that seems fairly well established is that it isn't simply the sheer bulk or fiber in it because other fiber-rich foods, Dr. Malinow points out, do not protect monkeys when they are fed cholesterol. One possibility is that alfalfa substances known as saponins, which form insoluble complexes with cholesterol, carry it through the intestinal tract so that it can't be absorbed.

A study on alfalfa and the blood fats cholesterol and triglycerides (high levels are a risk factor for heart disease) had positive results—7 people who took alfalfa seeds for 3 weeks had a big drop in their blood fats.

Amino Acids ★★★

"**D**rinking a glass of milk before you go to bed will help you sleep better."

Like many folk remedies, this homespun insomnia cure is based on scientific fact. Milk does the trick because it contains the amino acid tryptophan, a natural sleep-inducing substance. But tryptophan and many of the other amino acids—the so-called building blocks of protein—can do a lot more for you.

Tryptophan. This amino acid aids your body's own natural regulator of sleep, serotonin. According to Ernest Hartmann, M.D., who is a professor of psychiatry and a sleep researcher at Tufts University School of Medicine in Boston, 1 gram of tryptophan was enough to shorten sleep latency (time needed to fall asleep) by 30 to 50 percent in the normal subjects and mild insomniacs that he tested.

Best of all, tryptophan is safe—unlike the hypnotic drugs often prescribed for sleep problems. "Tryp-

tophan is rapidly metabolized and cleared by the body," wrote Dr. Hartmann.

But that's not the end of tryptophan's benefits.

"Tryptophan is a precursor of serotonin, a neurotransmitter in the brain, which potentiates the activity of endorphins (your body's own natural painkillers)," explains Samuel Seltzer, D.D.S., director of the Maxillofacial Pain Control Center at Temple University School of Medicine in Philadelphia.

In one trial of tryptophan's pain-killing powers, Dr. Seltzer started by testing 30 volunteers (all healthy and pain free) for pain perception and pain tolerance thresholds. "We used a special gadget that imparted an electrical current to the nerve of the tooth. As the voltage was slowly increased, the volunteers would signal when a sensation of pain was first perceived (pain perception threshold) and again when the pain became unbearable (pain tolerance threshold)."

The volunteers were then divided into two groups. One group was given tryptophan tablets and told to take one at breakfast, midmorning, lunchtime and midafternoon, and two before bedtime (a total of 2 grams per day).

The other group was given a dummy pill, or placebo, and was told to follow the same regimen.

"At the end of the experiment," Dr. Seltzer reports, "we again tested the volunteers for their pain perception and pain tolerance thresholds. The results were fascinating." In both the placebo group and the tryptophan

Is a craving for chocolate really a hunger for love? That's a question posed by Michael Liebowitz, M.D., of the New York State Psychiatric Institute, who found that romantic break-ups often lead to longings for chocolate. The link, he theorizes, is that romantic feelings produce phenylethylamine, a substance that's also in chocolate (phenylethylamine is derived from phenylalanine, an amino acid).

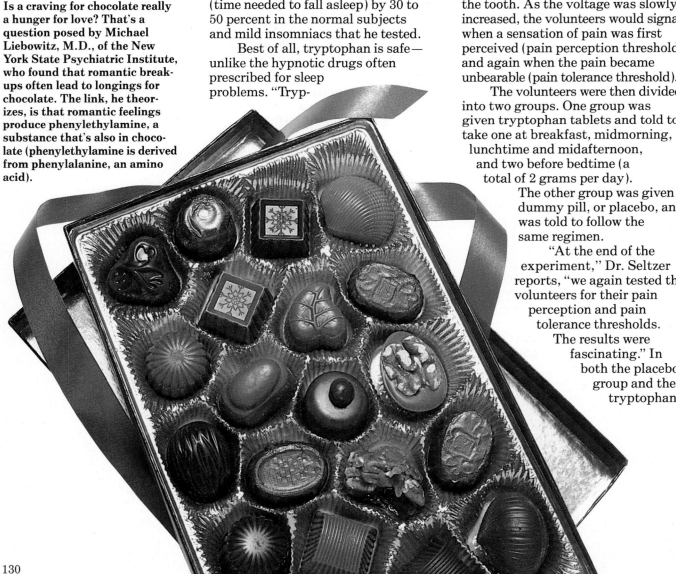

group there was no change in pain perception—when the volunteers first noticed pain. But 86 percent of the tryptophan group significantly increased their pain tolerance threshold.

Phenylalanine. This amino acid has been used to fight mental depression. In a study done at Queen Charlotte's Maternity Hospital in London, researchers found that some patients with depressive illness seem to be unable to produce enough of three substances known as trace amines. Because the body makes those amines from phenylalanine, the researchers suggest that phenylalanine supplements may help depression.

In addition, phenylalanine has been used to fight Parkinson's disease. In one study, all but 2 of 15 patients suffering from the disability and depression of the illness were able to "walk away" from some of their problems after four weeks of supplementation with a special form of phenylalanine. In another study conducted at the National University of Buenos Aires, 7 of 13 patients with walking difficulties showed "excellent" improvement—in fact, all of the patients improved somewhat. (People with PKU—phenylketonuria, a metabolic disorder that results in an excess of phenylalanine—should steer clear of phenylalanine treatment because they have an abnormal intolerance to it.)

Tyrosine. Still other studies have shown that the amino acid tyrosine can have a tranquilizing effect similar to phenylalanine's. A 30-year-old woman had suffered from severe depression for several years. Treatment with drugs only made her worse. But when a team of doctors from Boston and Cambridge, Massachusetts, gave her tyrosine supplements, her condition improved markedly after only two weeks.

Arginine. Finally, the latest news about amino acids—some news which may turn out to be the *best* news. The amino acid called arginine has been shown to stop the growth of cancerous tumors.

"In Japan, arginine water is sold as a health drink," notes Yoon Sang Cho-Chung, M.D., Ph.D. In her own work as chief of the cellular biochemistry section of the laboratory of pathophysiology at the National Cancer Institute in Bethesda, Maryland, Dr. Cho-Chung has found that arginine helps "straighten out" breast cancer cells.

"The breast cancer cells become flatter and enlarged—more like a normal cell," Dr. Cho-Chung explains.

Dr. Cho-Chung believes arginine may be involved in the body's production of cyclic AMP, a growth-regulating substance found in every living cell. Cancerous cells contain less cyclic AMP than healthy cells, and Dr. Cho-Chung has found that treating breast tumor cells with cyclic AMP helps to halt their growth.

Simply treating the cells with arginine will also help stop the cancer growth, but Dr. Cho-Chung gets the best results when she uses cyclic AMP and arginine together. "The tumor-inhibiting effect is enhanced, even if we use an amount of cyclic AMP that is ineffective when used alone," Dr. Cho-Chung explains. "We have found that we can lower the dose of cyclic AMP if we use arginine."

Since research into amino acids is so new, there are some slight cautions to taking them as supplements. First, if you have liver or kidney problems, don't take them at all. Second, if you take tryptophan by itself for four months or longer, have your doctor test you for the presence of indican, a potentially harmful substance that can form when tryptophan is metabolized by intestinal bacteria. Third, the best way to take amino acids—even if you're trying to get just one—is as a group in a multiple amino acid supplement. However, if you use a single amino acid, don't take it for one to two hours after you've eaten a protein like meat or milk; it won't be absorbed as well. And remember that amino acids are natural substances with little potential for harm. As one nutrition expert says, "They are mostly safe. There's nothing to worry about— except their cost."

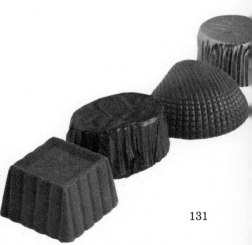

Bee Pollen ★

Bee pollen is actually *processed* pollen, pollen that bees have mixed with honey or nectar and then fermented in the hive. This so-called bee bread is the tiny animals' main source of nutrition. Apparently, it's the bee's knees to a bee, and that's why many humans claim it ought to be a be-all and end-all supplement for us.

But is it? Though a question that seems simple to answer—simply find out what's in the stuff—this one is a toughie, because our information is unreliable. Bee pollen, say its promoters, is about 20 percent protein, but in actuality, samples vary greatly. It also contains vitamins, minerals, enzymes, amino acids, fructose, glucose and lecithin. So much stuff, in fact, that the bee pollen advocates insist that it is the one food that has *everything* we need.

Who are these advocates? A good many are athletes. Lots of world-class runners, for instance, swear by bee pollen; they say that it allows them to run faster, run farther and regain their energy more quickly after a race. In addition, they report that bee pollen helps protect them from colds and pollen allergies, thus allowing them to compete more often.

Anybody else? Some folks with even smidgens of scientific credentials? Well, lots of apparently well-qualified researchers in Eastern Europe and the Soviet Union claim to have successfully treated anemia, obesity, rickets, diarrhea, skin problems and even mental illness with pollen. Unfortunately, only a few attempts have been made in the United States to verify or duplicate bee pollen's energizing abilities. In one recent study at Pratt Institute in New York, bee pollen was shown to improve endurance and speed; a placebo had no effect.

That's the good news in the pollen business. On the bad news side, bee pollen has been known to *cause* allergic reactions in people who are sensitive to all pollens. Of course, it may be that bacteria, mites, pesticides and bits of bee or other insects that become trapped in this product cause the problem, but it exists nonetheless.

Then too, there is the question of which type of pollen to use: the stuff straight out of the hive, or a type that's been commercially processed. The variety that's closer to its natural state is encased in a hard shell that seems impervious to the forces of nature and the ages. Archaeologists have found undamaged pollen buried in soil strata that are millions of years old, and so it's a real question whether pollen can be broken down by the human digestive juices alone. Commercially processed pollens, for their part, are subjected to all sorts of patented cleaning and packaging operations before they're sold. Some brands even manage to go directly from the flower to the package and somehow bypass the bee. What these industrial steps (or the absence of a bee) do to the nutritive value of the pollen is not known. Are these commercially processed pollens better or worse than the straight-from-the-hive varieties? Are they safer for people with allergies? Advertising claims aside, no U.S. studies on the subject have come up with convincing answers.

These worker bees nourished their queen (center) with royal jelly, a secretion from their salivary glands that supplied her with nourishment at birth. (She must like it; she lives about 13 times longer than they do.) It's no surprise that the substance is touted for its antiaging properties and is included in cosmetics to keep skin young. It's even used as a hair restorer. But don't get your hopes up. Sure, you'll pay royally for the product, but scientists say it's a pretender—it probably doesn't work.

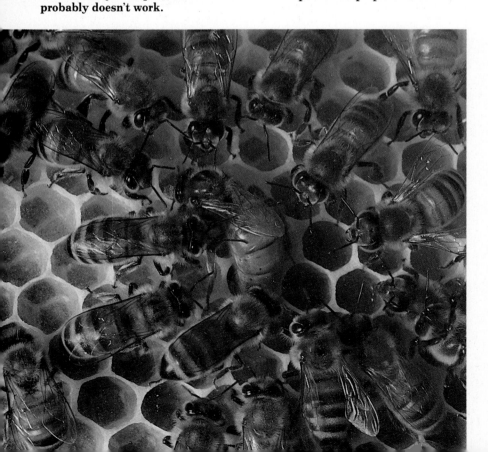

Brewer's Yeast ★★★★

It's a food! It's a food supplement! Who cares? It's *so* rich in *so* many basic nutrients that lots of experts have stopped trying to describe brewer's yeast and have simply taken to recommending it. But it's still a little ironic that nutrient-rich brewer's yeast comes out of the same vats as nutrient-poor beer. Brewers use yeast to ferment barley and hops into beer, but you should use it as a concentrated source of B vitamins, minerals and high-quality protein. This wonder yeast contains thiamine, riboflavin, B_6, B_{12} and folate. Plus, it's 40 to 50 percent protein by weight, contains very little fat and is a rich source of several important minerals—iron, potassium, calcium and, perhaps most important, chromium.

Besides adding this all-purpose nutrition to our lives, brewer's yeast also works directly to fight two major health problems: diabetes (especially the type that strikes older people) and cholesterol-induced heart disease.

Diabetes represents a failure of the body's system of carbohydrate metabolism. People with the disease have trouble regulating the use of the glucose (blood sugar) produced from the carbohydrates they eat, and they may require injections of insulin to do the job. But scientists are finding that the dependence of some patients (those with adult-onset diabetes) on insulin can be decreased, even eliminated, through the manipulation of their diet. These researchers have found that rats with problems of sugar metabolism were helped when brewer's yeast was added to their diets, and they determined that it was the trace mineral chromium doing the trick. Chromium is chemically linked to a combination of niacin and amino acids in a way that helps it increase the effectiveness of the body's own insulin in regulating blood sugar levels.

Chromium's benefits apply to humans as well as to rats. In one demonstration of that fact, scientists at Columbia University worked with elderly people, some of them diabetic and some of them not. The volunteers were fed either chromium-rich

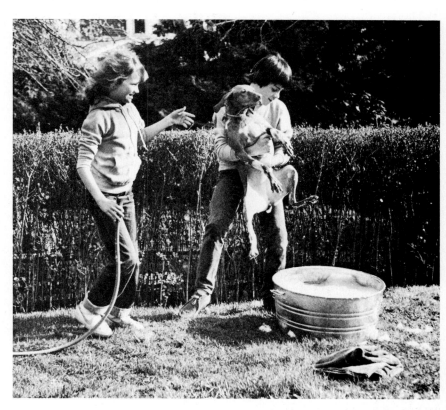

brewer's yeast or chromium-poor torula yeast as a supplement to their diet. The brewer's yeast improved sugar metabolism, not just in the diabetic patients, but in all the people tested.

On a second front, brewer's yeast also looks like a strong weapon in the fight against cholesterol and heart disease. J. Clint Elwood, Ph.D., a professor of biochemistry, and his colleagues at the State University of New York, Upstate Medical Center at Syracuse, studied the effect of brewer's yeast on serum cholesterol.

In the first trial, volunteers were instructed to take 20 grams (about 2 tablespoons) of brewer's yeast each day for a total of eight weeks. After the eight weeks, blood tests revealed that the cholesterol levels of the group had decreased significantly, says Dr. Elwood. The average decrease for all subjects was 10 percent, but a few of the volunteers had truly dramatic reductions in their total cholesterol levels. One dropped by approximately 110 points, while another decreased by 100, placing them both within a normal range.

Bathing your dog is one way to control fleas—but it's not good to do it more often than every 2 months because it dries out the skin. Brewer's yeast, however, can be used often and easily. Rubbed into a dog's fur, it works like flea powder, without the possible toxic effects of commercial products.

Even better, use brewer's yeast to build your dog's *inner* resistance to pests by adding it to his food. This rich source of B vitamins can make your pet healthier, says Richard Pitcairn, D.V.M., Ph.D., a nutritionally oriented veterinarian from California. A truly healthy animal doesn't get fleas.

Dr. Pitcairn suggests a dose of 1 tablespoon of brewer's yeast daily for every 50 pounds of your dog's weight.

Charcoal ★★★

What we're talking about here is more precisely known as "activated charcoal," and knowledge of its curative powers is not new. Ancient Egyptian healers used charcoal to treat poisoning and dizziness. Today, however, the substance is being used by scientists to combat skin infections, diarrhea, flatulence, hiccups and hangovers.

How does it work?

By being the most powerful *adsorbent* known to us. (An adsorbent is a substance that attaches things to its surface rather than absorbing them into itself.) Charcoal has the uncanny ability to adsorb nearly anything it contacts. Marjorie Baldwin, M.D., of the Wildwood Sanitarium and Hospital in Wildwood, Georgia, says it's like "a football field-sized piece of tissue paper rolled up into a tiny ball."

With that in mind, Raymond Hall, Ph.D., an associate professor of physiology at the Loma Linda University School of Medicine in California, pitted charcoal against intestinal gas. For the study, he selected 30 men and women, aged 18 to 40, and fed them a bland, non-gas-producing meal and measured intestinal gas generated over an eight-hour period. "The next day," Dr. Hall says, "we fed them a meal high in gas-producing foods—beans, whole wheat toast, peaches and fruit juice. For this meal, however, we divided them into two groups and gave one group activated charcoal capsules and the other placebos."

The group receiving placebos, says Dr. Hall, produced large amounts of gas. But the group receiving activated charcoal produced much less—*no more, in fact, than after the bland meal.*

"Activated charcoal reduces the amount of gas either by adsorbing the gas itself or adsorbing the intestinal bacteria that cause the gas," explains Dr. Hall.

But no matter how it works, Dr. Hall believes activated charcoal is "a good cure for gas. If a person has a gas problem, it's worth trying."

To ensure the best results, Dr. Hall suggests taking activated charcoal shortly after a meal. But, he emphasizes, activated charcoal won't quickly clear up a case of gas that's already developed. "It takes several hours for activated charcoal to reach the lower intestinal tract where the gas is being produced," he says.

Doctors in England have also used charcoal to treat infections. A letter to the medical journal *Lancet* described the use of charcoal-saturated cloth for wounds that were infected, discharging and had a bad odor.

The doctors applied a single layer of the charcoal cloth to the wounds of 26 patients with chronic leg ulcers and 13 patients with unhealed surgical incisions. "A noticeable reduction in wound odor occurred in 24 ulcer patients and 13 surgical wound patients," the doctors wrote.

Charcoal may solve still another annoying (albeit minor) problem— hiccups.

"I have treated my cases of hiccups with charcoal tablets," wrote a doctor to the *British Medical Journal,* "and have instructed patients to continue chewing them at least once an hour and in extreme cases continuously. In most cases I have met with success on this simple regimen."

Black Magic for Hangovers

Hangovers are caused by substances called congeners, and activated charcoal adsorbs them. In an experiment conducted at Columbia University College of Pharmaceutical Sciences in New York City, researchers asked 68 volunteers to drink either 2 ounces of whiskey, which has a high level of congeners, or 2 ounces of charcoal-filtered vodka, which has almost none. When the scientists measured hangover symptoms the next day, they found that 25 percent of the whiskey group had stomachaches, 27 percent had bad breath, 9 percent had dizziness and 6 percent had fatigue, while only 2 percent of the vodka group had headaches or upset stomachs, and there was no bad breath, dizziness or fatigue. Does that mean taking charcoal tablets before a night on the town could prevent a hangover? No one knows for sure, but it's possible.

Chlorophyll 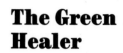 ★★★

The health benefits of chlorophyll, the green coloring agent found in plant leaves, have been the subject of much study over the years because of the close similarity that exists between chlorophyll and hemoglobin, the blood pigment in man. Like hemoglobin, chlorophyll consists of a web of similar molecules that are grouped around a single molecule of metal. In the case of hemoglobin, the metallic element is iron; in chlorophyll, it's magnesium. Small wonder chlorophyll has been referred to as "the blood of all plant life."

But despite the promising uses of the substance in areas like dental health, the prevention of both internal and external infections and even the control of cancer, much chlorophyll research remains speculative. To put this green therapy on a more practical footing, we offer the words of a nurse who has found dozens of practical uses for this "green blood." Meet Kay Haraguchi, R.N.

"Several years ago, I happened to come across an out-of-print article on chlorophyll in a friend's office, and I began experimenting with it on myself.

"One fall evening, while making candied apples, I accidentally burned myself when two drops of the boiling candy mixture landed on the middle finger of my right hand. Three weeks later the small burns, while no longer painful, were still open and unhealed.

"Then I remembered chlorophyll. Using a cotton swab, I dabbed a full-strength solution on the burns morning and evening. The results were amazing. I could literally watch the new tissue growing in from the edges of the wounds, and within five days both were completely healed.

"Another way I have used chlorophyll successfully is in a mouthwash. Oh, its green color will stain the basin, but it is easily washed away, and worth the effort. After I'd been using it for about six months, my dentist remarked that my gums, usually prone to inflammation, were much healthier. When I caught a cold, I tried gargling with chlorophyll and found that my sore throat seemed to disappear more rapidly."

Ms. Haraguchi is an occupational nurse at a large industrial plant near her home. She often finds uses for her chlorophyll remedies at work, especially for burns.

"The first-aid crew who were handling minor injuries before I came were using an anesthetic burn cream. It eased the pain of minor burns but did nothing to promote healing. I searched through pharmacies, wholesale drug houses and health food stores for a compound containing chlorophyll and could not find one on the market. So I mixed the soothing ointment with some chlorophyll, some vitamin E and a gel form of tannic acid, making an ointment one of the workers named 'Green Goddess Dressing.'

"The mixture proved itself. I knew I had a hit when the swing shift first-aid man requested a supply for each welder to keep in his tool box. He reported he'd found that if it was applied immediately, the minor burns welders got from brushing against hot metal did not form the usual blisters.

"A worker sustained first- and second-degree burns on a forearm when some burning oil accidentally ignited his shirt. I first cooled the burned tissue with an ice-water bath, then cleaned it with a germicidal soap. The burn compound was applied and the arm bandaged. For 10 days I changed the bandage daily, washing the arm each time before bandaging it with the ointment. Healing was complete in 14 days, with hardly any scarring.

"Of course, I never used this ointment on more serious third-degree burns, as the accepted treatment is to cool the burn, wrap it in sterile bandages and get the injured person to a hospital speedily.

"Another worker developed an ulcer just above one ankle. It was quite a painful affliction and had not responded to medical treatment. Every day for two weeks I cleaned the ulcer with hydrogen peroxide. Then I would apply liquid chlorophyll and vitamin E squeezed from a capsule onto the wound, and a sterile dressing. By the third week the ulcer was healed."

The Green Healer

Kay Haraguchi's burn cream combines 1 ounce commercial anesthetic cream, 1 ounce chlorophyll, 1 ounce tannic acid gel (all these ingredients are available, without prescription, from a pharmacy), 10,000 I.U. vitamin E and 2 drops iodine (as a preservative).

This mixture should be applied to first- or second-degree burns that are not extensive, and only after they have been cooled with ice or cool water. A bandage will be necessary because it is a gooey mixture. Mild burns should require just 1 application; more severe ones may be treated twice daily for 2 or 3 days.

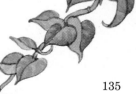

Desiccated Liver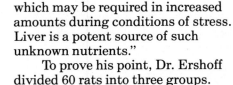

Desiccated liver is simply dried liver. (To desiccate, says Webster's dictionary, is "to preserve by drying.") The method of drying is unusual, however. The connective tissue (and in most desiccated liver products, the fat) is removed from beef liver, which is then dried in a vacuum at a temperature of about 140°F. In the process, 4 pounds of whole liver are required to make 1 pound of desiccated liver.

As a result, desiccated liver is a concentrated, convenient source of many of the nutrients that are provided by whole liver, with all of their health-building properties intact. That's doubly true, because the liver is the crossroads of metabolism and a storage point for nutrients, particularly iron.

But desiccated liver is also the source of an unidentified antistress factor. This elusive nutrient was closely studied by Benjamin Ershoff, Ph.D., a researcher who has written over 170 scientific papers. Several years ago, Dr. Ershoff wrote, "In addition to the known nutrients, substances are present in our diet which may be required in increased amounts during conditions of stress. Liver is a potent source of such unknown nutrients."

To prove his point, Dr. Ershoff divided 60 rats into three groups. He fed the first group regular laboratory chow, the second group the same chow supplemented with B complex vitamins and the third group standard chow with desiccated liver added.

He then made the rats from all three groups swim in a barrel of cold water until they were totally exhausted. The rats from the first group lasted an average of 13 minutes in the icy barrel. The second group did no better. But almost all of the rats on desiccated liver continued to swim for two hours.

Few of us are forced to swim in cold water, but like it or not we all undergo our share of stress in various forms: cranky children, irritable spouses, cars that won't start in the morning, leaky water pipes at home, jammed photocopiers at the office. (If anything can go wrong, it will . . . remember?) So to withstand all that stress, desiccated liver is ready, willing and able to supply that antistress factor touted by Dr. Ershoff.

Desiccated liver may also have special abilities to keep our gums in the pink. Harry Roth, D.D.S., formerly chief of periodontics at Beth Israel Hospital in New York, reports the case of a 19-year-old man who had incredibly inflamed gums. In fact, his whole mouth was unbearably sore and his tongue burned, to the extent that he couldn't tolerate acid foods like fruit or juices. After taking 21 tablets of desiccated liver a day, along with other nutritional supplements, for less than three months, all his symptoms disappeared.

Desiccated liver doesn't provide anything that you couldn't get from whole, cooked liver, of course. But it is low in one food factor that you'll be *happy* to get less of: fat. Desiccated liver has very little fat or cholesterol, which show up in fair amounts in whole liver. So desiccated liver is a useful source of nutrients for dieters or those people who are cutting down on cholesterol.

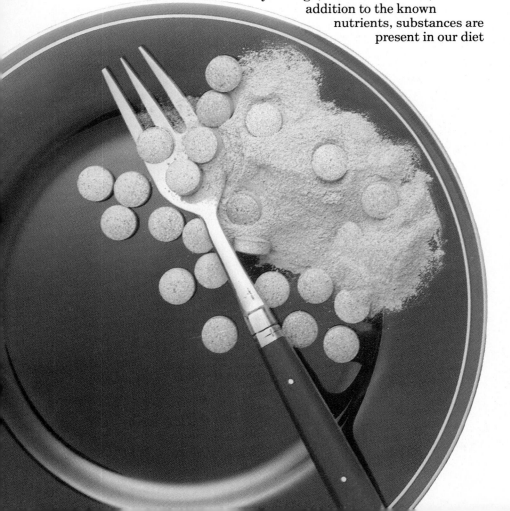

If you can't stomach the taste of liver but want its health benefits, you could try desiccated liver—a dried, concentrated form of the meat that comes in tablets or in powdered form (shown here out of the capsule).

Evening Primrose Oil ★

Evening primrose is a wild plant adorned by a long spike of yellow flowers that open in the evening. The seeds, which are about as small as mustard seeds, contain an oil that, like safflower and sunflower oils, is a valuable source of polyunsaturated fats, which are just as vital to health as vitamins and minerals. What makes primrose oil exceptional, though, is that it's the richest natural source of an essential fatty acid, gamma-linolenic acid (GLA, for short). The only other substantial source of GLA is mother's milk.

GLA is precious because it stimulates the body to manufacture prostaglandin E1 (PGE1), a hormone-like substance present in every organ. PGE1 plays a key role in the round-the-clock function of these organs and influences cell repair and immunity.

The body can manufacture GLA from another essential fatty acid with a similar name, *linoleic* acid. But several factors can—and do—block that critical conversion of linoleic acid to GLA—and ultimately, to PGE1. One is a diet high in saturated fats like butter and cream. Margarine and other overly processed vegetable oils, often found in baked goods, also block the process. So does drinking a hefty amount of alcohol. Viral infections, cancer, a lack of insulin (as in diabetes) or an inadequate intake of zinc, magnesium or vitamin B_6 also interfere with the manufacture of GLA. Last, elderly people cannot convert linoleic acid to GLA.

Taking GLA in the form of primrose oil can make up for factors that prevent its formation in the body. Much of the research on the use of primrose oil has been fostered and carried out by David F. Horrobin, M.D., Ph.D., a British-born Canadian doctor, formerly a professor at the University of Montreal and now head of a research foundation set up expressly to study GLA reactions—or lack thereof.

"It has been suggested that lack of this key reaction may be a critical factor in the aging process, since it can explain many of the changes which are characteristics of aging, including damage to the cardiovascular system, the deterioration of the body's defense system and the susceptibility to cancer," says Dr. Horrobin.

None of those areas has been studied extensively, though. Scattered evidence merely *suggests* that because the GLA in primrose oil stimulants prostaglandin E1, it may protect against blood clots, arthritis, schizophrenia and multiple sclerosis and boost our ability to recover from stress.

Dr. Horrobin, however, claims the evidence *is* strong that primrose oil helps circulatory problems.

"We have found that people who have high blood pressure or high cholesterol start off taking four, six or eight capsules a day," says Dr. Horrobin. "It usually takes two to four months to bring things down to normal." After that, they take half or one-third as much.

For less cataclysmic problems, like eczema and brittle nails, there is more clear-cut evidence of primrose oil's benefits. Evening primrose oil was given to 17 children and 15 adults who had had allergic eczema for six months or longer. Each adult received two capsules twice a day (a total of 4 grams) for three weeks, then took placebos for three weeks. The children took half those amounts. All improved significantly during primrose oil therapy, reported Dr. Horrobin and his colleagues in the *Lancet*.

In another study, individuals who took two capsules of primrose oil along with vitamins B_6 and C (two nutrients that may help activate primrose oil in the body) three times a day, solved long-standing problems with brittle, splitting fingernails.

Primrose oil is available in gelatin capsules. The few doctors who've studied primrose oil usually recommend four to eight capsules a day, half in the morning and the rest at night.

What makes this weed special? It's evening primrose. And though it's so common it may be growing in your backyard, its *seeds* are unique. They're 1 of only 2 natural and substantial sources of gamma-linolenic acid (GLA), an oil some scientists say can do wonders for your health.

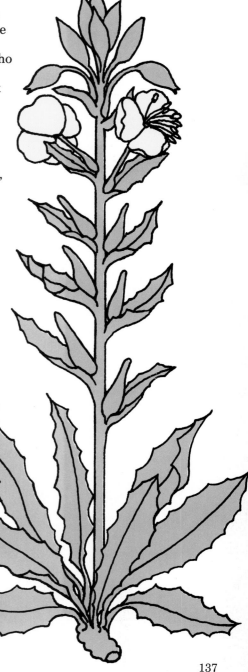

Fish-Liver Oil ★★★★

Cod-liver oil (the most common form of fish-liver oil) is one of Mother Nature's vitamin supplements, supplying large amounts of vitamins A and D. Ounce for ounce, cod-liver oil provides over 10 times more vitamin A than spinach, almost 8 times more than carrots and over 30 times more than apricots or broccoli, all good sources of the vitamin. It also provides over 200 times more vitamin D than vitamin D-supplemented milk, over 30 times more than egg yolk and over 650 times more than beef steak. Vitamin D enhances calcium absorption and prevents the bone deformities of rickets and (in adults) osteomalacia. Unless you live in a warm climate and soak up lots of sunshine, fish-liver oils are your most dependable source of vitamin D.

But cod-liver oil contains more than vitamins. It also contains a remarkable fatty acid: eicosapentaenoic acid (EPA). Scientists have found that EPA cuts down the tendency of blood to clot. That means cod-liver oil may prevent thrombosis, the formation of dangerous blood clots responsible for many heart attacks and strokes, as well as phlebitis (a blood clot in the leg) and other painful conditions.

And as little as 5 teaspoons a day of cod-liver oil will do the trick, according to a study by J. H. Brox and colleagues at the University Hospital of Tromso, Norway. EPA levels rose—and blood-clotting tendencies went down—in ten healthy men who took daily supplements of cod-liver oil for six weeks.

EPA also protects against heart problems by lowering cholesterol. In one study, people who took cod-liver oil every day for 12 days had a 13 percent drop in their cholesterol levels. The oil was discontinued for a short time and then resumed for a second 12-day period. At the end of the second period, cholesterol levels had dropped 17 percent below the levels prior to the experiment.

The heart-saving properties of EPA weren't always as apparent as they are today. Identified by a team of scientists from Aalborg Hospital and the Wellcome Research Laboratories in Denmark, this fatty acid seems to be the missing piece in a puzzle researchers have sought for years to solve: Why is it that Eskimos of northwest Greenland are much less likely to suffer coronary diseases than people in industrialized countries?

Past studies on Eskimos' blood lipids (fats) have shown excellent patterns for heart health—low levels of cholesterol, triglycerides and

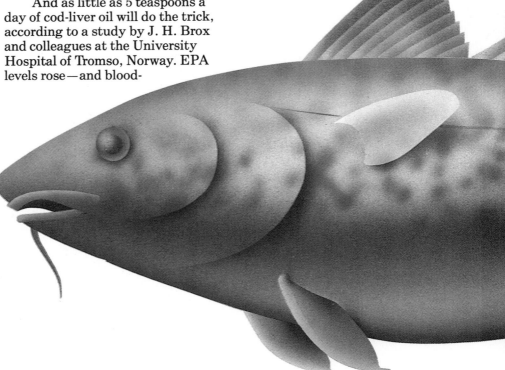

low-density lipoproteins (LDL), and high levels of the artery-clearing high-density lipoprotein (HDL) cholesterol.

How do the Eskimos manage to have such good blood lipid patterns? Is it a legacy from their aboriginal ancestors? Apparently not. Eskimos living in Denmark and eating like the Danes do not show the same healthy blood lipid patterns as the cousins they left behind in Greenland, reported the group of Danish doctors. In fact, Eskimos living in Denmark showed even *higher* cholesterol and triglyceride levels than the Danes whose civilized diet they very likely swallowed with a vengeance. Yet, when the researchers compared the composition of the Greenland Eskimo diet and the average Danish diet, they found that the Eskimos were consuming almost twice as much cholesterol as the Danes. Why were blood cholesterol levels of Greenland Eskimos much lower?

In the Eskimo diet, the main source of protein is meat. But this meat originates from animals living in the sea. The special polyunsaturated fatty acid in which the Eskimo diet and blood lipids are so rich is found primarily in certain arctic

types of fish. According to data compiled by Georg Lambertsen and Olaf R. Braekkan of the Government Vitamin Laboratory and the Norwegian Fisheries Research Institute in Bergen, Norway, medicinal cod-liver oil is a rich source of this factor.

Along with protecting against heart disease, cod-liver oil may also soothe arthritis. Charles Brusch, M.D., a medical director of the Brusch Medical Center in Cambridge, Massachusetts, gave 98 arthritis patients cod-liver oil every day for six months. Ninety-two showed major clinical improvement. "The majority of our patients," reports Dr. Brusch, "evidenced increased warmth in their extremities, less swelling and more energy after four or five months."

Dr. Brusch says that he has been recommending cod-liver oil to his arthritic patients for many years. He advises patients to take 2 tablespoons of cod-liver oil mixed with 2 tablespoons of fresh orange juice or cool milk.

If you don't care for the taste of the liquid, cod-liver oil also comes in clear, tasteless capsules.

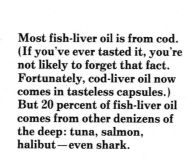

Most fish-liver oil is from cod. (If you've ever tasted it, you're not likely to forget that fact. Fortunately, cod-liver oil now comes in tasteless capsules.) But 20 percent of fish-liver oil comes from other denizens of the deep: tuna, salmon, halibut—even shark.

Ginseng and Glandulars ★

The official botanical name for this herb is *Panax ginseng,* *panax* coming from the Greek word *panacea,* or cure-all. Sadly, it's *not* an all-purpose remedy. But science *is* giving ginseng a serious look, along with some grudging compliments.

The ingredients that probably are responsible for ginseng becoming the most widely used herb in Oriental medicine's repertoire of tonics and restoratives—and which have gotten modern Occidental researchers interested—are glycosides. According to Stephen Fulder, Ph.D., in his book, *About Ginseng* (Thorsons Publishers, 1980), these dozen or so glycosides "are not very different from some of the hormones of the body."

The glycosides may be responsible for the warm feeling that accompanies ginseng's action as a stimulant. (It is as a stimulant that ginseng is best known and most widely accepted.) "It can be taken for tiredness and exhaustion," claims Dr. Fulder, "or when going through heavily taxing tasks, such as examinations, long-distance driving, stage performances, unusually strenuous physical work and so on."

Ginseng is alleged to be great for a long list of ailments. Nevertheless, there's little evidence that that's the case. In fact, no specific disease can be said to be cured by ginseng.

While ginseng is a generally safe (if not astonishingly effective) herb/drug, it does occasionally present real health problems. It has a tendency to elevate blood pressure significantly in some people, and thus should be avoided by those with high or borderline high blood pressure. There also seems to be a so-called ginseng abuse syndrome—high blood pressure, nervousness, sleeplessness, skin eruptions and morning diarrhea—that afflicts some regular users.

A PILL FOR THE GLANDS

Patients with hypothyroidism (an underactive thyroid) used to be routinely given a glandular product—dried pork thyroid. A daily dose, replete with the gland's hormones, somehow could spark the thyroid into action.

Synthetic chemical equivalents have almost completely replaced the real thing, but nonprescription glandular and organ extracts (namely adrenals, thymus, spleen and intestines) are still available. Presumably, if you have weak adrenal glands (which control body chemistry), taking a bit of animal adrenal gland will help you out. Or if you have colitis, taking whole animal intestine may help patch things up.

Unlike thyroid extract, however, those glandulars were never widely used by doctors, even though dozens of medical studies were done during the 1930s and 40s on the use of various glandular extracts and organ extracts for health disorders.

"The results were promising, but never followed up," says Jonathan V. Wright, M.D., of Kent, Washington. "The question remains as to whether the body actually uses glandulars, breaks them down, or passes them out unused.

"I use glandulars occasionally," continues Dr. Wright. "But frankly, I never know whether they're going to work or not—which is exactly what I tell the patient. Sometimes they work, and sometimes they don't."

Ginseng roots like this one are big business—the U.S. imports nearly $6 million worth a year from the Orient. But in this case the balance of payments is in America's favor. $34 million worth is exported *to* the Orient, where folks think the American-grown variety is best.

Kelp ★★

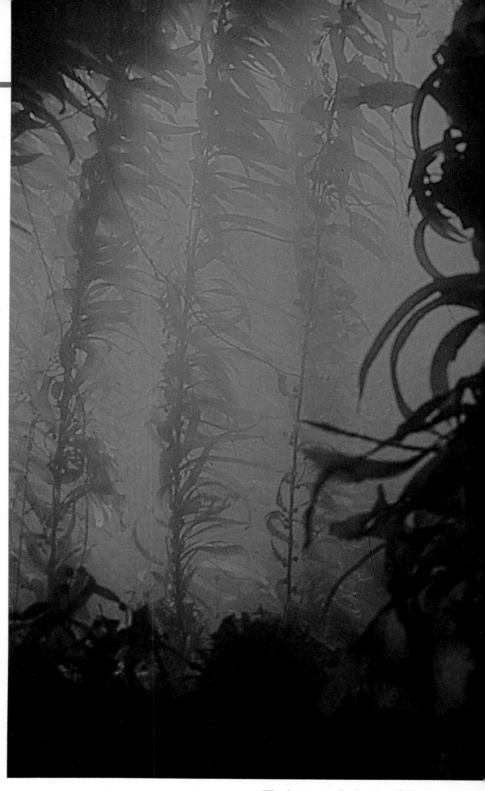

Kelp grows like a weed—a *sea* weed. Growing as much as an inch every hour, this brown alga snakes up from the ocean bottom, often growing up to 200 feet or more. To support that giant spurt of growth, the plant draws in an abundance of nutrients from the mineral-rich ocean.

One of those nutrients is iodine, a trace mineral ("trace" because only very small amounts are required for health) necessary for the prevention of goiter, a disease of the thyroid gland. In developing nations, goiter is still found in areas where people eat small amounts of seafood—but is a rarity among people who live near the sea and eat kelp.

Kelp is also a rich source of potassium, a mineral necessary for the health of the kidneys, heart and skeletal muscles. It also supplies some calcium, iron, zinc and magnesium. The vitamin content of kelp is as diverse as the mineral content. It provides small amounts of thiamine, niacin, riboflavin, and vitamins A and C.

Scientific reports show that kelp is valuable not only as a food but also as a medicine. Japanese folk medicine teaches that kelp can prevent and treat high blood pressure. And in a scientific study on kelp and high blood pressure, individuals fed kelp extract (algin) obtained relief from their high blood pressure symptoms.

Algin has also proved effective against heartburn. Researchers selected 60 patients with complaints of heartburn and acid regurgitation and divided them into three groups. One group received a placebo, another received an antacid and the third group received antacid *and* algin. All 60 patients took six tablets a day for two weeks. The number and duration of heartburn episodes were significantly reduced in the group receiving algin. Neither the placebo nor the antacid alone had a significant effect.

A form of algin—alginate—has also been used to prevent the intestinal absorption of radioactive strontium, one of the most hazardous substances generated by a nuclear blast. In a study, strontium was given to volunteers after they had received 10 grams of alginate. Twenty-six days later the strontium was administered again. Blood and urine tests showed that alginate had reduced the uptake of strontium.

Using kelp is simple—it can be cooked and served like spinach. It is available as a supplement in tablets and capsules. And, in powdered or granular form, kelp can be sprinkled from a shaker and used as a seasoning.

The farmers who harvest kelp don't have to worry about a meager crop—the huge sea plant can grow 2 feet a day.

Lecithin ★★★★

ecithin is a unique fatlike substance combining various factors such as the mineral phosphorus and the nutrient choline. Found in the lining of every human cell, it performs numerous roles in the maintenance of health.

In the brain, the choline in lecithin is transformed into acetylcholine, a chemical compound that relays information from one nerve cell to another. In the liver, lecithin metabolizes fat. In the bloodstream, lecithin helps prevent fats from accumulating on the walls of the arteries. And in the intestinal tract, lecithin enhances absorption of vitamins A and D and possibly the other fat-soluble vitamins E and K.

Lecithin reacts with fat by forming an emulsion, droplets in which two substances that normally do not combine are mixed. Fat and water are two such substances. Lecithin emulsifies them. Because it is an emulsifier, lecithin is often used commercially as an ingredient in margarine, ice cream, chocolate and other products.

Manufacturers usually select soybean lecithin for this purpose (lecithin is found in human,

Multiply this single soybean plant as far as your mind can stretch to get a picture of the U.S. soybean crop: about 136 billion pounds in just 1 year. About one-tenth of 1 percent of that is used to manufacture lecithin.

animal *and* vegetable cells). But soybean lecithin is not only used commercially; it is also useful medically.

"Lecithin has a long history," says David Kritchevsky, Ph.D., biochemist and associate director of the Wistar Institute of Anatomy and Biology in Philadelphia. "It's been in the medical literature for at least 30 years. We know that lecithin can actually reverse atherosclerosis in animals if it is injected. But people can't walk around with needle tracks all over their arms. So we keep experimenting with lecithin orally in people and in animals."

And the findings of these experiments are very encouraging. In one study, a group of people with high cholesterol had eaten a low-fat diet for over a year but still showed little change in cholesterol levels. They were given 2 tablespoons of lecithin three times a day. After three months, 12 of the 15 had major reductions in their cholesterol level.

In another study reported in *Current Therapeutic Research,* 21 patients with high levels of cholesterol and/or triglycerides were given lecithin supplements for 120 days. In 11 of 17 patients with high cholesterol and 8 of 12 with high triglycerides, levels returned to normal.

More important, lecithin shows a remarkable knack for changing the proportions of HDL cholesterol and LDL cholesterol. "The more HDL relative to LDL you have, the lower your chances of getting coronary heart disease; the less HDL, the greater the likelihood," says Dr. Kritchevsky. And lecithin not only reduces total cholesterol, it also increases the proportion of HDL to LDL—thereby preventing artery problems.

In a study conducted by Dr. Kritchevsky, rabbits that had high cholesterol and atherosclerosis were fed a controlled diet that included 1 percent lecithin. Although their atherosclerosis was not reversed, their HDL relative to LDL climbed 60 percent.

Other researchers have noticed the same effect in people. At Rutgers Medical School, researchers studied the effects of feeding 30 grams of lecithin for 16 weeks to 12 people who had elevated cholesterol with coronary artery disease. Lecithin raised the HDL factor, prompting the researchers to conclude that lecithin may exert "a favorable effect" against atherosclerosis.

At the University of Washington in Seattle, 12 people with normal cholesterol levels took 36 grams of lecithin for five successive three-week periods. Their HDL increased by an average of 3.6 percent, and their LDL decreased by 7 percent.

And combining lecithin with a prudent diet—low in fat and alcohol—works even better.

Ronald K. Tompkins, M.D., of the department of surgery, UCLA School of Medicine, conducted a study of four men and one woman, 64 to 84 years of age, in which they took 48 grams of lecithin per day for 24 months. In addition, they reduced their fat intake to 50 grams per day and their cholesterol to 300 milligrams and ate no fried foods or those high in saturated fats. "The entire group showed a decrease in cholesterol values during the low-fat and lecithin combinations," says Dr. Tompkins. Indeed, the average drop in cholesterol was 22 percent.

In Sweden, five 50-year-old men took 1.7 grams of lecithin per day for nine weeks, also abstaining from alcohol. Their HDL went up an average of 30 percent.

In a similar study in Italy, 21 people with elevated cholesterol took 1.8 grams per day of lecithin, drank no alcohol and cut down on their intake of saturated fats. More than 92 percent of the people with elevated LDL returned to normal levels.

"The present results," said the researchers, "underline the therapeutic value of [lecithin] in [people with elevated cholesterol]."

Lecithin may also help several kinds of brain diseases in which

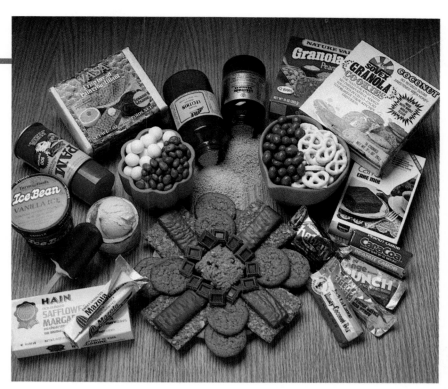

acetylcholine metabolism is abnormal. Five conditions—Huntington's chorea, tardive dyskinesia, Gilles de la Tourette's syndrome, Friedreich's ataxia and Alzheimer's disease—have all shown some improvement when patients received lecithin.

Lecithin may also dissolve or reduce the size of gallstones. Doctors gave lecithin and another substance to nine gallstone patients. In three patients, the gallstones shrank or dissolved completely.

Soybean lecithin is sold as a liquid, in liquid-containing capsules and in granular form. The granular form is the most concentrated, 1 tablespoon equaling approximately ten 1,200-milligram capsules in lecithin content. Granulated lecithin can be taken as is, or sprinkled in soups or salads, added to gravies, sauces or dressings or mixed in juice or milk drinks.

What do all these foods have in common?

Lecithin.

It's there as an emulsifier. Some substances just won't mix (like oil and water), but lecithin binds them together by dispersing tiny droplets of one substance in a drop of the other. So when you see "lecithin" on labels, don't worry—it's not an additive you have to be afraid of.

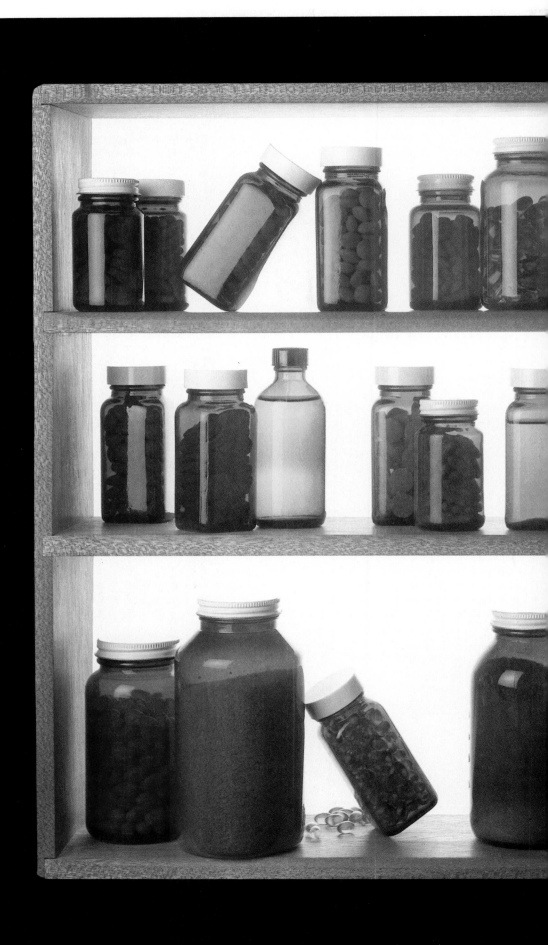

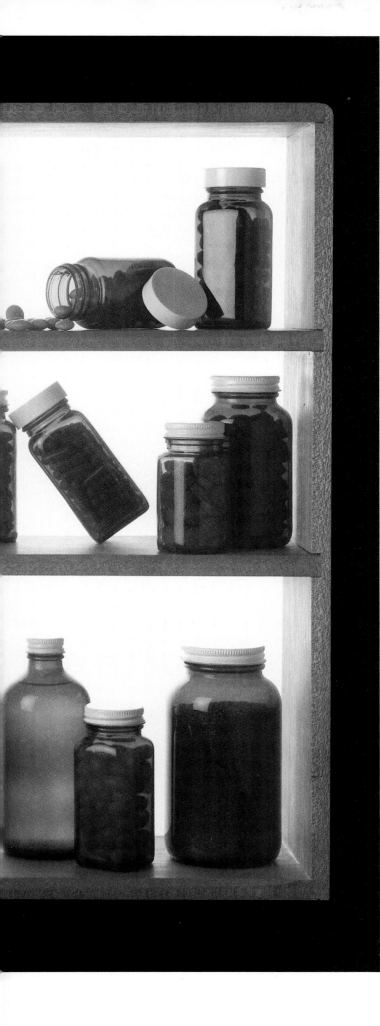

A Shopper's Guide to Supplements

Expert advice to help you choose supplements that are good for your body—and your budget.

There you are in the health food store or supermarket, standing in front of seemingly endless shelves stocked with every vitamin and mineral known to man. The bottles of vitamin A alone take up a space as wide as a truck. And even in picking one nutrient, you're confronted with *choices*.

Product 1 is "organic." Product 2 is in a "natural base." Product 3 lists the same potency as Product 4, only it comes from fish oil. Product 5's special feature is that it's in a "timed-release capsule." And Product 6 promises to deliver everything that Product 5 does— only at a lower price because it's *not* timed-release.

Shopping for food supplements can be *very* confusing. But two hints can help you through the maze. First, your supplementation program should be geared to your *individual* needs. If you want to take 5 milligrams of B_6, for example, don't buy a supplement with 50 milligrams of all the B vitamins.

Second, remember that the companies that manufacture food supplements are in business— their product labels combine equal amounts of sales pitch and fact. Make a practice of reading labels carefully so that you buy what you need instead of a high-priced pill stuffed with questionable extras (more about those "extras" in a moment).

But reading labels isn't as simple as it sounds. Some of the words look like they just hopped off the page of a science textbook; others (like "organic" or "natural") have been used so often in so many different ways that you're not sure just what they mean.

To help you out, we talked to pharmaceutical and nutrition experts who have their label terminology down cold. On the pages that follow are the definitions of some of the more common

Timed-release vitamins are usually more expensive than regular brands because they're designed to make sure you absorb more of the nutrient. Design is one thing, fact is another. This study of vitamin C showed that timed-release capsules were low man on the absorption totem pole, topped by 3 other kinds of vitamin C supplements: a regular tablet, a chewable tablet and vitamin C crystals dissolved in water.

terms. For convenience, we've arranged them in alphabetical order.

Buffered. This term is usually found on vitamin C products. The most common form of vitamin C is called ascorbic acid, which might be hard on people with sensitive stomachs. (The "acid" here is not the type found in sulphuric acid or other nasty chemicals, but the acidy tang of a lemon or lime.) The buffer mutes the acid a bit, making it gentler on digestion. A vitamin C product labeled "ascorbate" is also of the buffered variety. If you're watching your salt intake, avoid sodium ascorbate.

Emulsified. You'll find this term only on the oil-soluble vitamins, A, D and E. Oil soluble simply means that in the body the vitamins dissolve in oil, not in water; because of this, they're easily stored in organs like the liver, where they can be tapped when you need them. When these vitamins are emulsified, they also dissolve in water, making them more easily digestible by people who have a

tough time digesting oils or other fats.

Enzymes Added. Enzymes are substances that are found naturally in the digestive tract; they help break down food. If a supplement contains enzymes, the principle is that the enzymes will help break down the supplement so that you'll absorb the nutrients better. But if you take your supplements with meals (and you should), those enzymes are manufactured by your body; paying extra for them is like paying a tax on breathing. There are, however, some people who might benefit from enzyme-containing supplements: those who've had digestive tract surgery or who have very poor digestion.

Organic. The word "organic" tells you about as much about a supplement as the word "dog" would tell you about a puppy you were thinking of buying. In short, almost anything can be called organic—and is. Since there's practically no government regulation on the term, manufacturers can slap it on products without

Vitamin C Dosage Form	Timed-Release: Its Timing Is Off	Percentage of Dosage Absorbed
Timed-Release Capsule		14.2
Tablet		29.8
Chewable Tablet		30.4
Solution		32.1

thinking twice. Of course, some supplements *are* organic—which, in the strict sense of the word, means that they contain food concentrates that are chemical free and that are from food grown in soil that was never treated with pesticides, fertilizers and the like. But the fake products may have spoiled it for the rest, and you might want to avoid organic products if they're a lot more expensive than regular brands.

There is, however, an exception to this rule. In the case of some minerals, like selenium and chromium, organic (or "organically bound") means that the minerals were put into a yeast base, and those microscopic plants incorporated the mineral into their own structure. In this form, the mineral isn't over-absorbed by the body, which can happen if it isn't combined with yeast.

Timed-Release. Such supplements are supposed to dispense small amounts of a nutrient over several hours' time so that absorption stays at an even pace—levels don't go way up only to drop near zilch an hour or so later. The idea makes perfect sense—but the supplements only make money. As you can see from the graph on page 146, when it comes to absorption, timed-release products may be second rate.

WHAT ABOUT CHELATION?

Chelated minerals are a type of supplement product that has made a big splash in recent years. Chelate (pronounced key-late) is from a Greek word meaning claw: A chelated mineral is hooked up to another substance such as an amino acid. The supposed advantage of chelation is that the mineral is more usable by the body. Once again, the advantage may be more theoretical than real.

According to Richard M. Jacobs, Ph.D., acting chief of the FDA's nutrient toxicity section, "Chelation does not impart any nutritionally important advantage for mineral substances. Chelated minerals may be more *or* less available for use by the body than the mineral salts."

Explains Dr. Jacobs, "Their

usefulness is largely dependent on the tightness by which the chelator holds on to the mineral and the contents of the stomach when the chelate is consumed. For example, both zinc [gluconate] and copper gluconate are chelates with weak bonds. On reaching the stomach these bonds are quickly broken. Therefore these chelated forms would be equivalent to the salt forms of these minerals. So chelation usually makes little difference in how much we absorb. However, chelated minerals may be less irritating to the gastrointestinal tract as compared to some of the salts of these minerals when they are not consumed with a meal."

Which is *not* the way they should be taken, says Dr. Jacobs. Mineral supplements should be taken with meals, because food components—protein and carbohydrates—carry minerals into the system, in effect acting as the body's own chelators.

NATURAL OR SYNTHETIC?

The truth is, there's not much of a choice, because there's no such thing as a totally natural vitamin. But what about those labels that say "natural"—and those price tags that make you pay extra for it? What about all those claims that natural vitamins are better than synthetic—purer and more potent? Well, if you're taking natural vitamins, it's time to take them with a grain of salt. Here's why.

Most natural vitamins aren't a simple concentrate directly derived from a food source. They may *start* with food. But that food is processed in a very unnatural way. It's doused with harsh chemicals to eliminate unusable material; it's pumped with preservatives to keep it from spoiling; it's rolled and pressed and squeezed and stamped. These supplements are the natural end product of food about as much as a sheet of scented pink stationery is the natural end product of a tree.

And some manufacturers of natural vitamins don't bother with food at all. Their product is concocted in a factory just like the synthetic variety because it's too costly to do it any other way. So how do they get away with calling their brand natural?

The FDA, which regulates what vitamin manufacturers can and can't put on their labels, simply doesn't have enough manpower and money to check all the products whose labels say that they're natural. And

since "natural" is good for sales, a lot of companies exploit that lack of enforcement—and you.

Things the FDA does check, however, are content and potency. If the label says 500 milligrams of vitamin C, there had better be that amount of that specific vitamin in each tablet in the bottle. To make sure their vitamins are as potent as the label says, manufacturers of vitamin supplements that *are* natural (like yeast containing B complex vitamins), *add* synthetic vitamins to their products. It's so much cheaper to do that than to analyze the supplement to see if it meets the potency on the label.

Natural vitamin E is the exception. It's *all* natural. That is, if the E-rich goop that's left over from the processing of vegetable oil and then subjected to repeated chemical treatments and then colored so that you don't see the stuff floating in it (which can't hurt you but looks unappetizing) can be called natural, then there is such a thing as natural vitamin E.

True, a small percentage of natural vitamin E on the market is made from wheat berries and goes through minimal processing. But it's important to note that nearly every scientific study we know of that showed a health benefit from vitamin E (or any other vitamin) used the synthetic variety.

To sum up: No vitamin is truly natural. And even if it was, it wouldn't be better for you than a synthetic. What is different about the two kinds is their price; natural is often more expensive. And that's not healthy—for your budget.

Keeping Your Vitamins Fresh

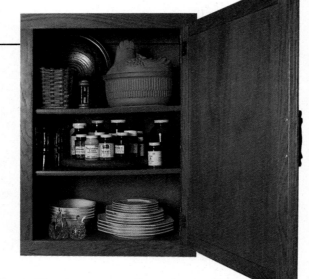

Most tablets and capsules last for at least 2 years without much loss of potency *if* you take proper care of them. For instance, don't leave them on the windowsill, where sunlight will speed their breakdown. And don't store them in the bathroom, where moist, warm air will do the same. Instead, stash your nutritional treasures in a closet or cabinet. (Not one over the kitchen sink; it's too moist there as well.) The air temperature in a closet stays cooler than that in a room, and closets also stay dry and dark.

As for storing vitamins in the refrigerator, it's recommended only if you live in a very warm, moist climate. If you must refrigerate your vitamins, be sure to bring them to room temperature before you open the bottle to prevent condensation from forming inside.

When you close the container, close it tightly. Loose lids expose vitamins to air and moisture. A final tip: If you plan to store your supplements for a long time, buy either single-vitamin capsules or all-vitamin (no minerals) supplements, because the presence of minerals may cause a faster rate of breakdown. As for minerals alone, they're tough as rocks.

HOW NUTRITION SCIENTISTS SHOP FOR SUPPLEMENTS

Vitamin A. Eli Seifter, Ph.D., professor of biochemistry and surgery at Albert Einstein College of Medicine, has conducted research showing beta-carotene (which turns into vitamin A in the body) may fight cancer. He says that we should try to get about 8,000 to 16,000 I.U. of beta-carotene (the amount in one sweet potato) daily from natural sources.

Synthetic or Natural: Is There a Difference?

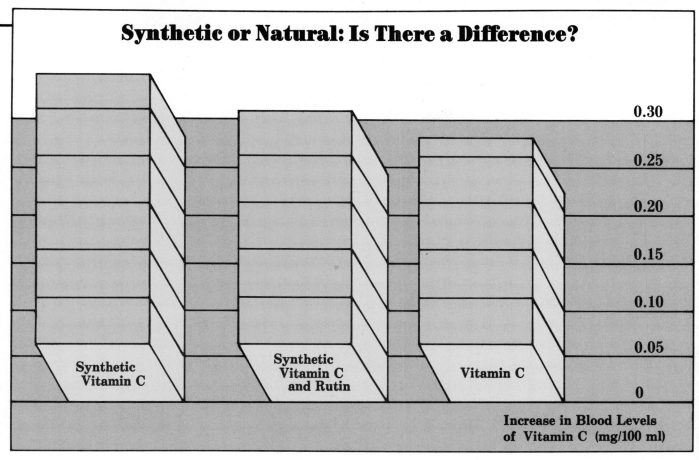

	0.30
	0.25
	0.20
	0.15
	0.10
	0.05
	0

Synthetic Vitamin C

Synthetic Vitamin C and Rutin

Vitamin C

Increase in Blood Levels of Vitamin C (mg/100 ml)

In addition, says Dr. Seifter, "I prefer a 10,000-unit supplement of vitamin A taken with a meal. I prefer the synthetic over the natural." (Natural vitamin A is derived from fish oils, but it's been processed so much that it can hardly be called natural anymore.)

"Natural vitamin A supplements contain vitamin D in varying amounts," he adds. "Unless the manufacturer tells you the amount of D in the product, I can't recommend it. We need only 400 I.U. of vitamin D daily, and some supplements contain too much." Dr. Seifter doesn't take supplements of vitamin D because he gets what he needs from milk, where "the vitamin is in the presence of what it helps absorb—calcium and phosphorus." However, he points out, people who live in cloudy places such as the American Northwest, or people who are shut-ins, need a multivitamin containing vitamin D.

B Complex Vitamins. We asked Roger J. Williams, Ph.D., D.Sc., of the University of Texas, discoverer of a member of the B complex, panto-thenate, about buying B complex

supplements. One tip he gave us is to "measure B supplements against food charts to be sure they contain at least the amount of B vitamins that are found in B-rich foods." (Use the chart in chapter 4.)

"I once saw a supplement of potassium which I later found equaled the amount of potassium in one lima bean," he told us.

Dr. Williams takes an "insurance" supplement of B in moderate quantities. In his opinion, although a B vitamin from a natural source might have extra unknown benefits, "a B vitamin is a B vitamin."

Vitamin C. "One should shop around and buy the cheapest form of vitamin C," asserts Linus Pauling, Ph.D., the two-time Nobel laureate and an advocate of vitamin C. "It's essentially all the same. I myself take ascorbic acid powder because it's the pure crystalline form and the least expensive. One level teaspoon contains about 4 grams of vitamin C." Dr. Pauling is not concerned about bioflavonoids (the nutrients that frequently accompany vitamin C in nature), although he does take his powdered C mixed in orange

One supposed advantage of natural vitamins is that they're better absorbed than the synthetic variety. This study showed otherwise. It tested the blood levels of vitamin C in people who took synthetic vitamin C; synthetic vitamin C with rutin, a bioflavonoid; and the natural vitamin C of orange juice. As you can see, the synthetic variety had the highest absorption rate.

juice, which has bioflavonoids.

Ascorbic acid pills are good, too, according to Dr. Pauling, but he cautions that ascorbic acid might "not be for those few people with sensitive stomachs." Calcium ascorbate is a good alternative.

Vitamin E. William J. Hermann, Jr., M.D., of the Memorial City General

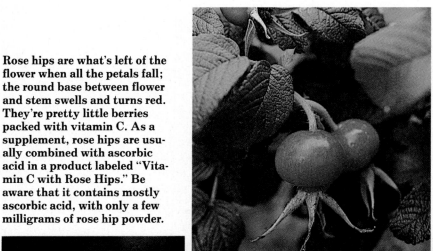

Rose hips are what's left of the flower when all the petals fall; the round base between flower and stem swells and turns red. They're pretty little berries packed with vitamin C. As a supplement, rose hips are usually combined with ascorbic acid in a product labeled "Vitamin C with Rose Hips." Be aware that it contains mostly ascorbic acid, with only a few milligrams of rose hip powder.

Hospital in Houston, found that vitamin E favorably altered cholesterol levels in his heart patients. The type he used? "A cheap synthetic variety," says Dr. Hermann. "I don't know if the natural form, d-alpha tocopherol, would have brought about different results. But we found the synthetic form [dl-alpha] very effective."

Actually, dl-alpha tocopherol is only one of eight chemical compounds, called tocopherols, that make up vitamin E. The other compounds include beta, gamma and delta. Some E supplements—labeled "mixed tocopherols"—include all of the compounds, but there's no proven advantage to having them all. In fact, research has not shown the particular value of any tocopherol other than alpha.

Calcium. Anthony Albanese, Ph.D., of White Plains, New York, has been remarkably successful in helping

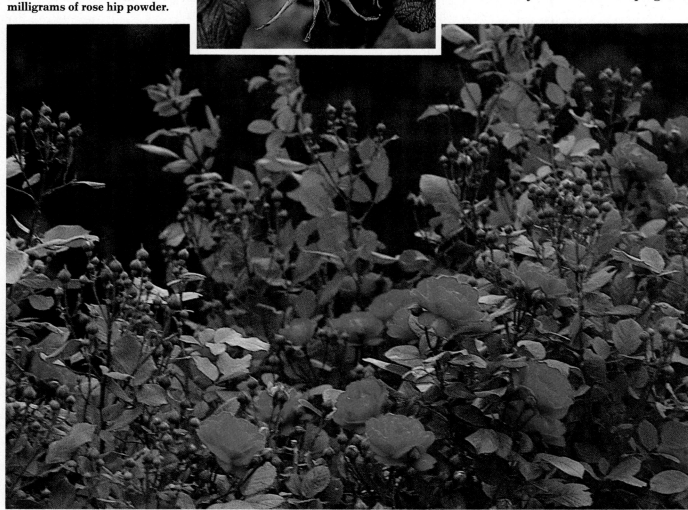

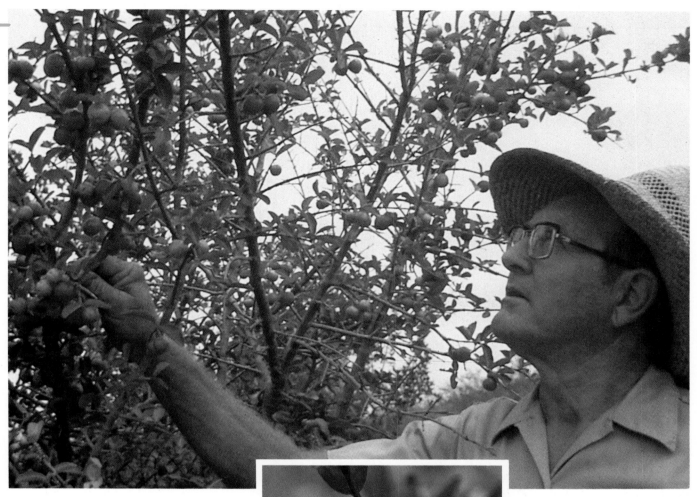

Acerola cherries, grown on trees in the warm climes of Barbados, Puerto Rico and Florida, are the richest natural sources of vitamin C—1,000 to 2,000 milligrams or more of ascorbic acid per 100 grams of juice. Making supplements entirely from acerola powder, however, is prohibitively expensive. "Vitamin C Acerola" supplements contain only tiny amounts of acerola. The rest is synthetic vitamin C.

reverse osteoporosis through calcium supplementation. "We restrict our treatment primarily to calcium carbonate," says Dr. Albanese.

"Over the years we have compared various forms of calcium, beginning with calcium gluconate. This made only 10 percent of the calcium available to the body, so we needed to give large doses and more pills. Too many pills are hard for older people to swallow. Calcium lactate and citrate were better, at roughly 20 percent. Then we tried calcium carbonate, which yielded 40 percent. We could give two to three tablets per day and meet our patients' needs." Dr. Albanese quit searching once he settled on calcium carbonate. "It's a relatively inexpensive source and not hard to come by."

Marvin Bierenbaum, M.D., of the Atherosclerosis Research Group, Montclair, N.J., who has shown that calcium carbonate lowers cholesterol, says, "Other types of calcium do not have the same effect."

Iron. Sean Lynch, M.D., professor of medicine at the University of Kansas,

confirmed what other experts say: "Soluble iron salt—that is, ferrous sulfate—is the best iron supplement. It's also the cheapest."

Zinc. "In most humans zinc is well absorbed from the gut regardless of the form," says Carl C. Pfeiffer, M.D., Ph.D., of the Princeton Brain Bio Center. "In practice, then, the cheapest salt of zinc is preferable. For the American market, this is . . . zinc gluconate."

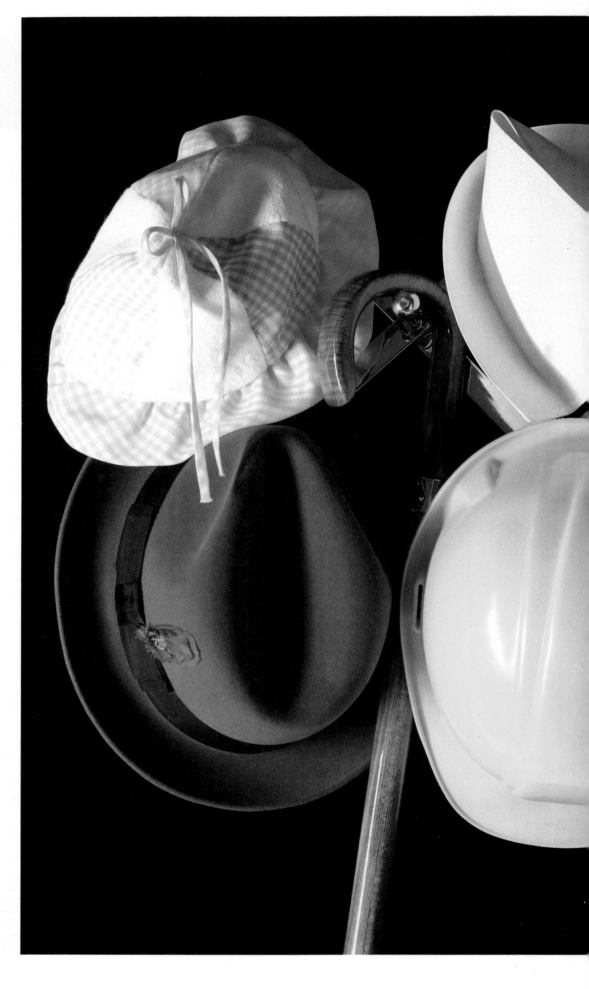

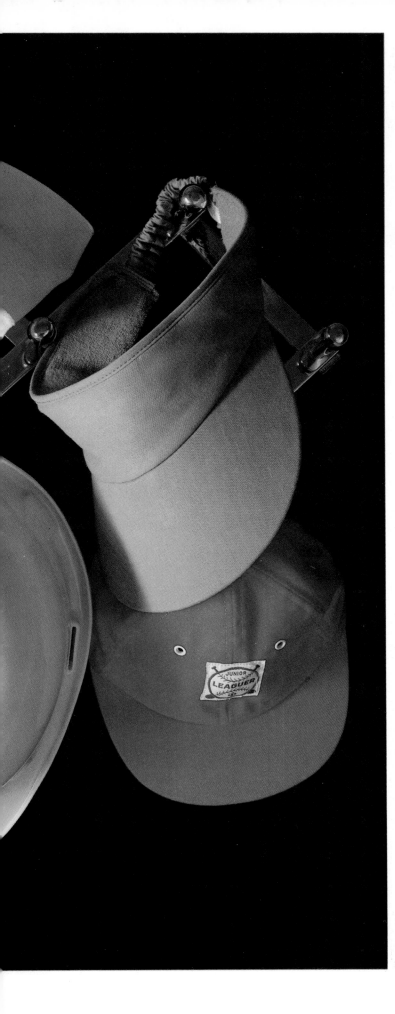

A Personal Supplement Program

This tailor-made nutritional guide shows how much of each vitamin and mineral *you* need.

Like the one-size-fits-all shirt, the typical multivitamin/mineral supplement is supposed to cover everybody—as though people were made in a mold. But scientific research has confirmed time and again that your nutritional needs are as individual as your fingerprints.

Roger J. Williams, Ph.D., D.Sc.—a research scientist at the Clayton Foundation Biochemical Institute, University of Texas—states in his book, *You Are Extraordinary* (Random House, 1967) that "each of us is built in a highly distinctive way in every particular, and this is the basis of individuality."

Dr. Williams coined the term biochemical individuality to describe this concept:

"Recognizing biochemical individuality, we can accept the fact that Winston Churchill violated many of the rules of good nutrition and lived magnificently in old age, without jumping to the conclusion that nutrition is unimportant for other individuals, including ourselves. Recognizing inborn differences in body chemistry will make commonplace the fact that some individuals should fear the use of alcohol while others have almost no chance of becoming addicted to it.

"If we continue to try to solve [nutritional] problems on the basis of the average man, we will be continuously in a muddle, because the concept of 'the average man' is a muddle. Such a man does not exist."

Michael Colgan, Ph.D., nutritional researcher and author of *Your Personal Vitamin Profile* (Quill, 1982) agrees with Dr. Williams: "Compared to the mythical textbook average, you may have inherited . . . low or high blood pressure, poor or keen eyesight, sharp or dull hearing, high or low sex hormones, sluggish or explosive thyroid and a zillion variations. The unique combinations are endless. And they require unique fuel. For optimum health you need a blend of nutrients different from anyone else's."

Biochemical individuality isn't the only factor that customizes your need for nutrients. If you smoke a pack or more of cigarettes a day, for example, your blood levels of vitamin C may be reduced by 40 percent. Women who exercise vigorously for 30 to 50 minutes a day may double their need for riboflavin. The physical stress of being ill can steal up to 60 percent of your body's vitamin A. And pregnancy increases a woman's needs for nearly all nutrients.

Can you meet these increased needs—not to mention your body's normal need for vitamins and minerals—by taking a nutritional supplement that supplies 100 percent of established Recommended Dietary Allowances? As we discussed in chapter 2, a growing number of physicians and research scientists don't think it's possible. Alan R. Gaby, M.D., a family practice physician in Baltimore, Maryland, points out that the RDAs are defined as "the levels of intake of essential nutrients considered . . . to be adequate to meet the known nutritional needs of *practically all healthy persons* [italics ours].

"Actually," says Dr. Gaby, "a case could be made that very few of us are truly healthy—that we are a nation of chronically ill people. One-third of us will develop heart disease; one out of five will die of cancer. Three of ten women will develop severe thinning of their bones after the reproductive years. Millions of men will suffer from prostate troubles as they get older. The millions who require medication for anxiety, depression or pain are also chronically ill. While our bodies are slowly developing these problems we should not be considered healthy, even though we may feel well. For if we were better nourished, the degeneration would probably proceed at a slower pace. It might even be prevented entirely.

"Another large group of people for whom the RDAs may not apply are the elderly," Dr. Gaby points out. As people get older, they lose the ability to absorb nutrients efficiently. As a result, nutrient needs become greater.

John Francis Catchpool, M.D., of Sausalito, California, believes that "RDA" is a misnomer. "As Linus Pauling has pointed out," says Dr. Catchpool, "it should be called the 'MDA', for *Minimum* Dietary Allowance, because if you take any less, you are a prime candidate for a deficiency."

So throw out that one-size-fits-all shirt and have your nutritional program tailor-made. Mind you, even such a customized system of nutrition can't be very exact. After all, the whir of changes in your environment, your diet and your body is ceaseless. And nutritional science is not yet geared up for high-precision calibration of anyone's vitamin and mineral needs. But it is possible to discover some measurements that should result in a reasonably good fit.

To that end, this chapter gives you two or three possible levels of intake for each nutrient. They're neither tools for the diagnosis of medical problems nor prescriptions, so don't try to use them as substitutes for professional medical care. But do consider them carefully. They represent a distillation of current nutritional research and may be your best bet for defining your personal vitamin and mineral profile.

Some of the nutrients covered in this book aren't included in the guidelines. The trace metals chromium and selenium, for example, are still in the initial stages of investigation and it's difficult to be precise about appropriate levels. We do know that a lack of chromium is associated with diabetes and heart disease and that some diabetics have been able to lower insulin requirements by taking chromium supplements under a physician's supervision. Likewise, a deficiency of selenium has been linked to a higher incidence of cancer. So someone who is at risk for cancer (a smoker, for instance) may wish to consult a nutrition-oriented physician to assess his dietary status for selenium.

Potassium, another nutrient not in the guidelines, is best obtained from food sources, although some physicians give supplements to patients especially low in the mineral.

Bioflavonoids, which were discussed at the end of chapter 5, aren't really vitamins, and it's difficult to be exact about how much you need. People who bruise easily or who have hemorrhoids might benefit from supplements, however.

It's also difficult to pin down your need for the B vitamins biotin and inositol, and for choline, a substance closely related to the B vitamins. But any B complex supplement you take should supply enough of all three.

As you read the guidelines, please keep in mind the following:

1. These guidelines are not specific recommendations, but rather general, informational statements.

2. For each nutrient, read the paragraph of descriptive statements accompanying the various amounts. *Find the paragraph that most closely describes you.* It is not necessary, or in some cases even possible, for each sentence in the paragraph to describe you specifically. Go with the one that, *overall,* seems most applicable.

3. Don't try to use the information here to pinpoint nutritional causes of symptoms. Analyzing serious symptoms is your doctor's job.

Nutritional supplements, especially in therapeutic doses, should be taken *only* on the advice (and with the supervision) of your physician. There can be serious physical effects resulting from supplementation, particularly in persons taking medication (for example, blood pressure levels may change in hypertensive patients taking calcium supplements) or in persons with special sensitivities to specific nutrients.

4. For your information, we have included some specifics on problems that crop up when a person takes too much of any one nutrient. Remember: *All* substances— even water and oxygen—are potentially toxic if taken in excess.

5. The list given is not complete. There are other vitamins and minerals, as well as special foods, for which regular intake may be advisable. However, the vitamins and minerals listed are commonly considered the most important, and there is enough known about them to be able to draw up these general guidelines.

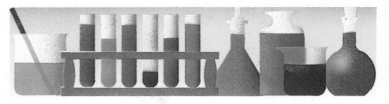

Does Hair Analysis Work?

When it comes to your total health picture, doctors need various readings on what your body has enough, too much or too little of. And when it comes to finding out a person's mineral status—especially levels of potentially poisonous heavy metals such as lead, mercury and cadmium —blood, urine and tissue samples simply can't show *cumulative* levels.

But hair can. Minerals and metals move from the body into hair in concentrations at least 10 times higher than in blood or urine. They are stored and trapped there, forming a permanent linear record, sort of like a ticker-tape. So, an analysis of hair can show not only recent but also long-term accumulations.

It's easy to get a hair sample: Just snip a spoonful or so, close to the head, near the base of the neck.

So far, so good. But once the specimen is sent to a laboratory to be analyzed, things sort of break down. First of all, hair dyes and permanent waves can fool analyzing tools into making false evaluations. Some shampoos, especially antidandruff shampoos, leave zinc or selenium residues on the hair. In addition, different labs use different methods of analysis and can come up with different results using the same hair. (The American Holistic Medical Institute has now published a set of test performance standards, but not all labs conform to them.)

On top of that, there are no standards of interpretation; 2 doctors could conceivably read the same printout results and interpret them 2 different ways. And hair analysis *is* tricky; certain minerals that show high levels in the hair may actually be deficient in the body. So a doctor needs lots of experience interpreting hair reports.

Hair analysis has a lot of possibilities. But right now it's not a great test for telling whether or not you have high levels of pollutants in your body. And anybody who tells you he can give you a total nutritional profile from this test is pulling the wool over your eyes.

VITAMIN A

"Deficiency of vitamin A is not only a major nutritional problem in many developing countries, but also in countries such as the United States and Canada. It has been well documented that [low vitamin A] results in an enhanced susceptibility of the respiratory system, bladder and the colon to chemical carcinogenesis."
—Zahid H. Siddik, Ph.D., National Cancer Research, Surrey, England.

5,000 I.U. Your diet regularly includes liver, carrots, broccoli, apricots, sweet potatoes and spinach. You are generally in excellent health, your resistance is very high and your environment is low in pollutants. Naturally, you are not a smoker. Nor are there any smokers in your household. There is nothing in your family history that makes you particularly concerned about cancer.

10,000 I.U. You eat vitamin A-rich foods such as liver, carrots and sweet potatoes occasionally, but they're not on your menu every day. Your health is better than average, but when your resistance gets low, you tend to become ill, perhaps with upper respiratory symptoms. Skin problems are not unknown to you. You are exposed to an average amount of pollution.

25,000 I.U. Occasionally, you notice patches of dry, bumpy skin on your legs or arms. Not dry and flaky, but dry and *bumpy.* Recently you may have had a serious health crisis such as surgery, an injury, a burn or other problem that had you out of circulation for a while. Your vision, especially at dusk, is not what it could be. Spinach and carrots have been known to appear on your dining table, but they are hardly fixtures.

Therapeutic Dosages. Normally, supplements of vitamin A should not exceed 25,000 I.U. per day. However, very large amounts (as much as 200,000 I.U.) have been used—under a physician's supervision—to treat severe skin problems (such as cystic acne) and severe eye problems (such as xerophthalmia). Too much vitamin A can be toxic; symptoms of excess include dry skin and loss of appetite.

THIAMINE (VITAMIN B₁)

"We studied a group of teens who complained of headaches, abdominal and chest pains and sleeping problems. They were irritable and some were aggressive and hard to handle. Our blood test showed them to be deficient in thiamine. We changed their diets and gave them thiamine supplements. Of the 10 we retested, all showed normal behavior."
—Derrick Lonsdale, M.D., Cleveland, Ohio.

5 Milligrams. You're practically famous for your perpetual good mood and unflagging energy. Your diet regularly includes brewer's yeast, wheat germ, whole grain products, nuts, liver and sunflower seeds.

10 Milligrams. You're generally a frisky sort, even though you aren't necessarily ready to conquer the world at the dawn of each and every day. There are times when you wish your nerves were better behaved, and you sometimes think you drink too much coffee or tea, or eat too many sugary foods, for your own good. Your diet is average.

25 Milligrams. Your nerves are definitely in a state, and you may be suffering from depression, loss of appetite or similar emotional and neurological problems. Your energy levels are at best undependable, as is your memory. Perhaps you enjoy more than just a few drinks more often than you should. Possibly you are in your retirement years, when absorption of thiamine—as well as other B vitamins—is reduced.

Therapeutic Dosages. Two conditions commonly treated with large doses of thiamine are the beriberi of alcoholics and Wernicke-Korsakoff syndrome, often brought on by chronic alcoholism. Therapy starts at 50 to 100 milligrams daily, via injection or intravenous solution at a hospital. Doctors also prescribe thiamine therapy for beriberi heart disease, schizophrenia and serious liver problems. The FDA states that the only adverse effects from large doses of thiamine occur in those few people who are hypersensitive to the vitamin. Physicians should check the status of *all* the B vitamins in patients receiving large doses of thiamine, in order to maintain a good nutritional balance.

RIBOFLAVIN (VITAMIN B₂)

5 Milligrams. You're a great one for dairy foods like milk, cheese and yogurt. Almonds, brewer's yeast, broccoli, liver, wheat germ, wild rice and other riboflavin-rich foods appear in your daily fare. Your eyes are clear and bright and the skin around your mouth is perfectly smooth—except when you smile, which you do frequently.

10 Milligrams. Milk and liver you don't care for, cheese has too much cholesterol for you and almonds and wild rice are too expensive. So you don't get that much riboflavin in your diet except from your whole grain bread. You are also getting up there in years.

25 Milligrams. If you look in the mirror carefully, you will see small cracks around your mouth, or your tongue may be smooth and purplish. Your eyes may burn, itch, be abnormally sensitive to bright light or simply feel worn out. You may feel depressed. You are no spring chicken.

Therapeutic Dosages. Extra riboflavin may be called for after surgery or injury since the vitamin is essential to normal growth and it helps repair body tissue. Thyroid disorders also demand more riboflavin. In hyperthyroidism, the body processes so much riboflavin that it becomes hungry for more, and in hypothyroidism, it processes too little.

For general deficiency disorders, as little as 10 milligrams daily usually clears up all symptoms, although much larger doses (around 75 milligrams or more) have been used by physicians for a severe deficiency involving riboflavin malabsorption. Excess riboflavin is excreted in the urine, so toxicity does not appear to be a problem.

> "The less riboflavin you have, the less you are able to utilize; once the body gets sick, it gets sicker, because it cannot utilize what little vitamin there is in the diet. . . . Riboflavin deficiency itself produces changes in the ability to utilize that same vitamin."
> —Richard Rivlin, M.D., New York Hospital-Cornell Medical Center.

NIACIN

10 Milligrams. Your diet regularly includes fish, beans, organ meats, peanuts, poultry, whole wheat products and brewer's yeast—or at least half of those foods. Your disposition is strictly blue sky. The only time you are irritable is when enemy tanks invade your neighborhood.

25 Milligrams. Your diet is nothing to brag about, and occasionally you wonder if there is some reason why it's becoming so difficult for you to fall asleep or if your headaches have some peculiar origin.

50 Milligrams. Your nerves and your personality are definitely not what they used to be and not what your friends or family would like them to be. You may have thought about visiting a psychologist or psychiatrist and you would be grateful if something could be done about your insomnia.

Your breath may be less than sweet smelling; in fact, it may be somewhat foul. In addition, your whole mouth feels sore and your gums are painful and possibly swollen.

Therapeutic Dosages. According to *Modern Nutrition in Health and Disease* (Lea & Febiger, 1980), a book by Robert S. Goodhart, M.D., and Maurice E. Shils, M.D., "the amounts of nicotinamide [a form of niacin] generally recommended for therapeutic purposes are about 10 times the daily minimum requirement . . . and range from 50 to 250 milligrams per day."

For pellagra, dosages range from 300 to 500 milligrams of niacinamide. Some doctors use niacin to treat schizophrenia. Amounts over 1 gram can cause nausea, elevations of blood sugar and uric acid and abnormal liver functions.

> "I think there is ample reason to believe that the amount of niacin a person should be getting for good health is not the amount most Americans are getting on a so-called normal diet. The diet is greatly shortchanged on all the water-soluble vitamins, and niacin is one of the most important."
> —Edwin Boyle, M.D., Medical University of South Carolina.

VITAMIN B₆ (PYRIDOXINE)

"In terms of performance or well-being, I think we could feel better than we do if we took vitamin B₆. A lot of people walk around fatigued from lack of sleep or overwork or stress. But with B₆, we might live closer to our potential . . . we could function at a higher level."
—John H. Richardson, M.D., Old Dominion University, Norfolk, Virginia.

5 Milligrams. You practically radiate good health, and your positive, energetic attitude is reflected in your intelligently varied diet, which includes brewer's yeast, brown rice, salmon, sunflower seeds, liver, bananas and broccoli.

10 Milligrams. You certainly aren't sick, but you sometimes wonder why your skin isn't better, or why your nerves aren't calmer. You may tend to retain fluid before your menstrual periods.

50 Milligrams. Your monthly period causes you considerable distress, not only because of fluid retention, but also because of mood swings, irritability and other emotional problems at that time—or perhaps *all* the time. Possibly you take birth control pills. Whether you are a man or a woman, life is looking more and more like an ordeal to you, and yet you can't

seem to pinpoint the cause of your depression.

Therapeutic Dosages. Some women with severe premenstrual syndrome may require large doses (500 milligrams) of B₆ before their period each month. The vitamin seems especially useful here when taken with magnesium. Pregnant women who suffer from morning sickness also respond well to B₆ therapy. And patients receiving chemotherapy may benefit from supplements of B₆, since their stores are depleted.

Large doses (200 to 600 milligrams per day) may decrease milk production in nursing mothers. Excessive doses (over 1,000 milligrams per day) may cause nerve damage. However, even small doses can interfere with the drug L-dopa (used for Parkinson's disease).

VITAMIN B₁₂

"Vitamin B₁₂ deficiency has been found to be common among elderly patients. [Blood] vitamin level profiles of noninstitutionalized elderly have shown 31.5 percent of them to have [low levels of] B₁₂ in the blood."
—David Martin, M.D., Falk Clinic, Pittsburgh.

5 Micrograms. You are healthy, energetic, haven't yet reached retirement age, and you regularly eat animal foods such as liver, beef, fish or chicken.

10 Micrograms. You've passed your sixtieth birthday and your ability to absorb this vitamin in a useful form may be on the wane.

25 Micrograms. Lately, your energy level and possibly your nerves just haven't been up to snuff. Possibly you've been ill or had surgery. You may be a strict vegan, a vegetarian who avoids all animal-source foods. Your symptoms may well be serious enough to suggest a thorough medical evaluation.

Therapeutic Dosages. Injections of vitamin B₁₂ are not an uncommon treatment for people suffering from chronic fatigue and other symptoms

of B₁₂ deficiency such as mood changes, forgetfulness, mental confusion and depression. Severe deficiencies of B₁₂, resulting in anemia and nerve damage, can be due to a lack in the diet or improper absorption. The stomach secretes an "intrinsic factor," which binds B₁₂ to the intestinal walls, where it is absorbed. Some people lack intrinsic factor due to decreased gastric activity or gastrointestinal surgery; they must take either injections of B₁₂ or large amounts of B₁₂ pills under a doctor's care. The treatment for pernicious anemia, a very dangerous condition, is sometimes aggressive: One medical text advises injections of about 100 micrograms one to three times per week until the deficiency is corrected and then injections given once monthly. Treatment is usually for life.

FOLATE

400 Micrograms. You eat a lot of raw green vegetables such as broccoli, asparagus and spinach. You're a liver lover from way back. You are full of energy and retirement is something that's far in the future.

400 to 800 Micrograms. You must remind yourself that you should eat raw green vegetables more frequently, and you wish you were able to work out a way to eat beans, broccoli, asparagus, brewer's yeast, tempeh and whole wheat products more often than you do. Your health is about average.

800 to 1,200 Micrograms. Lately you feel as though you've been under considerable emotional stress, and you haven't been able to handle it as well as you should. Your nerves in general have been in such a state that you have given serious consideration to seeking some kind of help, whether it be medical, psychological

or even nutritional. You are over 70 years of age and therefore your absorption of folate is likely to be impaired. Possibly you have recently undergone surgery. Your doctor may have reason to believe you have folate deficiency anemia, which causes, among other things, inflammation of the tongue, digestive problems and diarrhea. (When taking folate supplements, always take vitamin B_{12} with them.)

Therapeutic Dosages. In *Mental and Elemental Nutrients*, (Keats, 1975) Carl C. Pfeiffer, M.D., Ph.D., says folate therapy "eliminates the anemia of pernicious anemia" but that vitamin B_{12} must be taken along with folate "to cure the neurological symptoms of the disease." Amounts higher than 5,000 micrograms may "produce muscle restlessness, myoclonic (muscle) jerking and, occasionally, seizures."

"Folate deficiency is probably the most common vitamin deficiency in man, especially among poorer populations. It results in anemia, with all the attendant signs and symptoms: pallor, lethargy and weakness."
—Myron Winick, M.D., Columbia University.

PANTOTHENATE

5 Milligrams. Getting your "three squares" a day is practically a religion in your life; liver is on the menu at least once a week, and you eat plenty of whole grains and drink milk every day. You start each day feeling energetic and cheerful. In fact, you may have more get-up-and-go than co-workers your age (and younger). You live in a low-stress environment like the country or a small, friendly town.

25 Milligrams. Like many Americans, you commute to work and by the time you get there, you need a breather from the traffic. But the pressures of the job close in quickly and before you know it, you've grabbed a cup of coffee and scheduled two meetings for the morning. You sometimes have trouble falling asleep at night, and you skip meals. Allergies sometimes bother you.

50 Milligrams. It's not just your imagination: You *are* looking ten years older than you should. You suffer from fatigue and insomnia. Hay fever makes your life miserable every allergy season, and on top of that it seems like you've almost always got a cold. Possibly your feet feel like they're burning, a symptom of pantothenate deficiency.

Therapeutic Dosages. Some doctors report that large doses (200 to 500 milligrams) are useful for people with severe hay fever. Also, pantothenate is used to treat postsurgical paralysis of the gastrointestinal tract, in which abdominal pain and gas are problems. Very high doses (over 10 grams) can cause diarrhea and water retention.

"It is apparent that raw foods supply adequate amounts [of pantothenate]. It is not apparent, however, that persons subsisting on refined, processed and canned foods will be provided with adequate amounts. The data cast doubt on the adequacy of the American diet for . . . pantothenate."
—Henry A. Schroeder, M.D., Dartmouth Medical School.

VITAMIN C

"If you want to live a life of reduced infection, if you want to promote healing and sharpen your immune system, if you want optimum triglyceride levels in your blood, you'll want a daily intake of vitamin C far above the RDA."
—W. M. Ringsdorf, Jr., D.M.D., University of Alabama, Birmingham.

100 Milligrams. You can hardly remember the last time you were ill. Your health is excellent, and your gums are clear, firm and never bleed. Your daily diet includes generous measures of such vitamin C-rich foods as broccoli, cabbage, melons, citrus fruits and green peppers.

500 Milligrams. You feel that your resistance must be maintained at a high level in order to keep you feeling your best. There may be some chronic health problem or stress in your life, such as a bad back, allergies or exposure to cigarette smoke. Your diet is not bad by a long shot, but does not supply the amount of ascorbic acid you feel you should get.

1,000 Milligrams. You are definitely susceptible to stresses such as infections, pain or skin problems. Possibly you are recovering from surgery, an injury or any other serious bout with illness. In the past, you have noticed that injuries or surgical incisions seem to heal very slowly. Your diet could be better, but it is difficult for you to eat raw foods high in vitamin C, because they tend to make your gums bleed. You may want to step down to a lower level of vitamin C supplementation when the health problem or crisis you are now undergoing disappears.

Therapeutic Dosages. Very large amounts of vitamin C (several grams daily) have been used for a wide variety of ailments: colds, low back pain, drug withdrawal, mental illness and cancer. Common side effects are upset stomach and diarrhea. Since vitamin C can increase the amount of oxalate in the urine, there is a slight risk that people who previously formed kidney stones will form another, but this risk can be reduced by taking vitamin B_6 and magnesium daily.

VITAMIN D

"Vitamin D status may be poor, even in healthy populations, and especially among women. Also, it seems that the dietary intakes of the elderly in the United States may be somewhat lower than the RDA."
—John Omdahl, Ph.D., New Mexico School of Medicine

0 to 100 I.U. You live in an area where the sun shines strong and bright, such as Florida or southern California. What's more, you move around quite a bit outdoors, so that sunlight strikes your body, thus causing your system to manufacture its own vitamin D. If you have a year-round tan, you probably don't need any supplemental vitamin D at all.

200 I.U. You live in an area such as Washington state, where a beautiful sunshiny day is a real event. You are not a big drinker of milk, which is fortified with vitamin D, usually at the rate of about 400 I.U. per quart. Occasionally, however, you do eat fish containing vitamin D, such as herring, mackerel, salmon, sardines or tuna.

500 I.U. You probably live in the northern United States, Canada or England, where, except for a few weeks in the middle of summer, intense sunshine may be as rare as rainbows. What's more, for one reason or another, you do not get very much exercise outdoors. Possibly, you have had a problem with your bones, suffering a fracture or pain.

Therapeutic Dosages. Rickets and osteomalacia ("soft-bone diseases") call for vitamin D therapy; some doctors use vitamin D to treat arthritic pains and osteoporosis. As a general rule, you should be in close contact with a physician if you're taking any dosage over 400 I.U. daily. That's because vitamin D is potentially very toxic. In large doses, it can cause dangerous levels of calcium in the blood, leading to calcification of the soft tissues and, eventually, possible death. Nausea, loss of appetite and weight loss are all symptoms of toxicity.

VITAMIN E

100 I.U. You are relatively young, in fine health, and you live in an exceptionally clean area, where there is remarkably little pollution.

400 I.U. You may have a health condition that may be prevented or improved with vitamin E, such as intermittent claudication (cramping of the calf while walking) or any one of a number of skin problems. The air you breathe, the water you drink and possibly the food you eat contain the usual amount of pollutants found in our modern world. Your diet contains a substantial amount of fats that are polyunsaturated, such as corn oil.

600 I.U. You may be concerned about a circulation problem and feel that the beneficial effect of vitamin E on blood elements is something that you want to take advantage of in full measure.

Therapeutic Dosages. Some physicians prescribe rather large doses, up to 1,400 I.U., of vitamin E as a preventive measure against circulatory and heart disease in patients prone to these conditions.

Usually, vitamin E is relatively safe; in one study by the National Institutes of Health, individuals taking up to 800 I.U. daily for over three years showed no signs of toxicity. People with a vitamin K deficiency (it may be caused by taking an anticoagulant drug or having no vegetables in the diet, and its symptom is an impairment of blood clotting) should avoid large doses of vitamin E, which could worsen the deficiency.

"There are times when extra vitamin E is required in order to counteract the effects of excessive oxidized fats on tissues. People who eat a lot of fried foods are particularly vulnerable [to circulation problems] because frying allows oxidation of fats to take place faster. What's more, a diet like that may be deficient in vitamin E, compounding the problem."
—J. C. Alexander, Ph.D., University of Guelph, Ontario.

CALCIUM

800 Milligrams. You are a man, and your diet normally includes substantial amounts of such calcium-rich foods as dairy products, tofu, salmon (with bones) and broccoli. You get a good bit of outdoor exercise and your health is excellent in almost every regard.

1,000 Milligrams. Your diet is not especially high in the calcium-rich foods mentioned above. You sometimes have a tendency to develop muscle cramping when you aren't performing exercise that might cause such a cramp. Your teeth may be causing you problems, or your gums. If you are a woman, you have nursed several children. You may also have begun to experience minor backaches. Your mother or your grandmother, when they were older, suffered from bone fractures or osteoporosis. You eat a substantial amount of meat, which promotes excretion of calcium from the body.

1,200 Milligrams. You have aching bones, such as in the lower back. You seem to be developing kyphosis (dowager's hump) and you are clearly not quite as tall as you once were. Recently you have suffered a broken bone. Perhaps you have been told by a doctor that you have osteoporosis. You may frequently suffer from cramps in the calf at night. Your nerves are irritable and you have pains for which your doctor has been able to find no obvious explanation. You may be taking steroid drugs, which cause calcium depletion.

Therapeutic Dosages. Many doctors treat postmenopausal osteoporosis with daily calcium doses above 1,200 milligrams. Problems from excess intake are very rare, only occurring in people who absorb extra-large quantities of the mineral—a condition a doctor would be able to spot.

"Just think of your bones as a reservoir. If your body uses its reservoir regularly over a long period of time, your bones are sapped of calcium. Women who experience regular calcium deficiency from ages 20 to 50 can lose more than one-third of their bone calcium during that period of time."
—Louis Avioli, M.D., Washington University, St. Louis.

IRON

"People aren't dropping like flies from iron deficiency. But if you're talking about optimum performance, no, we aren't getting as much iron as we should. With the amount of iron most of us are getting now, we're not going to feel as strong or as energetic or as alert as we could be."
—Paul Saltman, Ph.D., University of California, San Diego.

10 Milligrams. You are an energetic sort and have a hearty appetite as well. If you are a woman, you no longer have monthly periods. Or if you do, there is an extremely small amount of blood loss. Your diet regularly includes meat, liver, beans, leafy green vegetables, dried fruits and whole grain foods.

20 Milligrams. You are a woman who is still menstruating. Your appetite is not exactly ravenous, and there are many days in which you eat no meat. Perhaps you drink tea, which can interfere with the absorption of iron.

30 Milligrams. Your periods are heavy. Or perhaps you have had surgery recently or lost blood for some other reason. You have one or more of the many symptoms of iron deficiency anemia, which your doctor has told you are not caused by disease; weakness, easy fatigue, poor resistance, headaches and pale skin are among them. If this is the case, your doctor may recommend even higher amounts of iron for six weeks or more.

Therapeutic Dosages. Iron (the most effective form is ferrous sulfate) is used to cure iron deficiency anemias. Typically, physicians encourage anemic patients to eat more iron-rich foods along with vitamin C-rich foods to enhance iron absorption. According to Helen Andrews Guthrie, Ph.D., in *Introductory Nutrition,* "therapeutic doses may contain as much as 250 milligrams of iron."

In large amounts, iron can be extremely toxic. Vomiting, diarrhea, rapid heartbeat, shock, coma and convulsions are all symptoms of iron poisoning. Small children are the most frequent victims, so iron preparations should be kept out of their reach.

MAGNESIUM

"Until we can define, more precisely, how much magnesium is needed for health—maintenance at different ages and under different physiologic, pathologic, dietary and environmental conditions—it is better to provide more than less magnesium."
—Mildred S. Seelig, M.D., New York University Medical Center.

250 Milligrams. Your diet regularly includes generous amounts of soybeans, brown rice, peas, green leafy vegetables, nuts and whole grain products. You live in a hard-water area and don't have any use for a water softener, which means your drinking water contains fair to good amounts of magnesium. Your nerves are steady and you have no particular reason to be concerned about the health of your heart. You do not engage in endurance sports such as cross-country running or Nordic skiing.

If you are a woman, you count yourself in with millions of other women who suffer from a moderate degree of premenstrual tension, which can be greatly lessened (or even eliminated) by supplements of magnesium taken with B₆.

400 Milligrams. Your nerves often seem to be on edge. You may even notice a certain amount of muscular tremor. You are concerned about doing everything possible that may help prevent a heart attack, due to a family history of heart problems or indications that you are at risk for a heart attack. Possibly you are a heavy drinker, which creates a need for more magnesium.

Therapeutic Dosages. Magnesium supplements should clear up a magnesium deficiency, the symptoms of which include irritability, nervousness, uncontrollable muscle contractions and general loss of neuromuscular control. Alcoholics may find themselves with those symptoms, as may patients maintained on magnesium-free fluids for a long time or patients who have had long bouts of nausea or diarrhea. Magnesium can be toxic to people with kidney failure and to women who are taking a magnesium-containing drug for toxemia of pregnancy.

ZINC

15 Milligrams. You are in excellent health and your diet includes such dependable zinc sources as meat, liver, oysters, fish, wheat germ and nuts. When you do injure yourself for some reason, the wound heals quickly. Your vision in dim light is excellent.

25 Milligrams. You are concerned about the possibility of developing an enlarged prostate gland and want to do everything possible to try to prevent it. Your vision at night may not be all that it should be. You may have skin problems, or surgical incisions or injuries that have taken a long time to heal. Your resistance might need some beefing up.

35 Milligrams. You may have any one of a number of problems that might possibly be helped by extra zinc, such as enlarged prostate, a variety of skin problems or a very poor sense of taste. Possibly you have had surgery recently and heal-ing is proceeding very poorly. You may have acne, even though you are not an adolescent. There may be white spots on your fingernails, which can be a sign of zinc deficiency.

Therapeutic Dosages. Sometimes a pronounced lack of appetite is caused by low dietary zinc; the treatment is "2 milligrams of zinc sulfate per kilogram of body weight daily" to restore appetite and sense of taste, says the textbook *Introductory Nutrition* (C.V. Mosby, 1979). Zinc is also used to treat problems of stunted growth and underdeveloped sex organs. There have been reports, too, of zinc sulfate benefiting sickle cell anemia patients.

A dietary excess of zinc, which can occur from storage of food or beverages in galvanized containers, can lead to fever, nausea, vomiting and diarrhea. It can also cause losses of necessary iron and copper stores, which may result in anemia.

"Because zinc deficiency is common in hospital patients and is characteristic of many chronic disease states, this deficit is probably a major factor in poor tissue repair and prolonged hospital stays. Fortunately, healing problems . . . respond well to zinc sulfate therapy."
—Walter J. Pories, M.D., School of Medicine, East Carolina University.

Your Personal Supplementation Program: A Worksheet

To use this worksheet, read through the guidelines and select the intake level that's right for you. Then write it down under the correct vitamin, along with any notes— for example, "When I feel like a cold is coming on, increase vitamin C."

VITAMIN A	NIACIN	VITAMIN D
THIAMINE	VITAMIN B$_6$	VITAMIN E
RIBOFLAVIN	VITAMIN B$_{12}$	CALCIUM
	FOLATE	IRON
	PANTOTHENATE	MAGNESIUM
	VITAMIN C	ZINC

Source Notes

Chapter 1

Page 4

"The First Vitamin Experiment" adapted from "Feeding Experiments Illustrating the Importance of Accessory Factors in Normal Dietaries," by F. Gowland Hopkins, *Journal of Physiology*, July, 1912.

Page 5

"How the Japanese Scuttled a Deadly Diet" adapted from *The Vitamin Hunters*, by Albert von Haller, translated by H. F. Bernays and Judith Heller (Radnor, Pa.: Chilton, 1962).

Chapter 2

Page 14

"Canning: The Great Vitamin Massacre" adapted from "Effect of Commercial Processing on Nutrients," by Daryl B. Lund, *Food Technology*, February, 1979.

Page 15

"Percentage of People Getting Less Than the RDA for Vitamins and Minerals" adapted from "Problem Nutrients in the United States," by Eleanor M. Pao and Sharon J. Mickle, *Food Technology*, September, 1981.

Page 16

"Vitamin C Handcuffs Pollutants" adapted from "Should the Concept of the Recommended Dietary Allowance Be Altered to Incorporate Interactive Effects of Ubiquitous Pollutants?" by Edward J. Calabrese in *Medical Hypotheses* (New York: Churchill Livingstone, 1979).

Page 17

"Drugs: One More Reason Why We Need Extra Nutrients" adapted from *Nutritional Support of Medical Practice*, Howard A. Schneider, Carl E. Anderson and David B. Coursin, eds. (New York: Harper & Row, 1977).

Chapter 3

Page 23

"The Best Food Sources of Vitamin A" adapted from *Nutritive Value of American Foods in Common Units*, Agriculture Handbook no. 456, by Catherine F. Adams (Washington, D.C.: Agricultural Research Service, U.S. Department of Agriculture, 1975)
and
Composition of Foods: Dairy and Egg Products, Agriculture Handbook No. 8-1, by Consumer and Food Economics Institute (Washington, D.C.: Agricultural Research Service, U.S. Department of Agriculture, 1976)
and
Composition of Foods: Spices and Herbs, Agriculture Handbook No. 8-2, by Consumer and Food Economics Institute (Washington, D.C.: Agricultural Research Service, U.S. Department of Agriculture, 1977).

Page 25

"An Acne-Control Program" adapted from "13-cis Retinoic Acid and Acne" by H. Jones, D. Blanc and W. J. Cunliffe, *Lancet*, November, 1980.

Page 35

"Can Vitamin A Block Out the Majority of Cancers?" compiled from information from the American Cancer Society.

Chapter 4

Page 39

"The Best Food Sources of B Complex Vitamins" adapted from *Nutritive Value of American Foods in Common Units*, Agriculture Handbook No. 456, by Catherine F. Adams (Washington, D.C.: Agricultural Research Service, U.S. Department of Agriculture, 1975)
and
Pantothenic Acid, Vitamin B_6 and Vitamin B_{12}, Home Economics Research Report No. 36, by Martha Louise Orr (Washington, D.C.: Agricultural Research Service, U.S. Department of Agriculture, 1969)

and
Composition of Foods: Poultry Products, Agriculture Handbook No. 8-5, by Consumer and Food Economics Institute (Washington, D.C.: Science and Education Administration, U.S. Department of Agriculture, 1979)
and
Composition of Foods: Dairy and Egg Products, Agriculture Handbook No. 8-1, by Consumer and Food Economics Institute (Washington, D.C.: Agricultural Research Service, U.S. Department of Agriculture, 1976)
and
"Folacin in Selected Foods," by Betty P. Perloff and R. R. Butrum, *Journal of the American Dietetic Association*, February, 1977.

Page 47

"Losses of B_6 in Processing" adapted from "Losses of Vitamins and Trace Minerals Resulting from Processing and Preservation of Foods," by Henry A. Schroeder, *American Journal of Clinical Nutrition*, May, 1971.

Chapter 5

Page 59

"The Best Food Sources of Vitamin C" adapted from *Nutritive Value of American Foods in Common Units*, Agriculture Handbook No. 456, by Catherine F. Adams (Washington, D.C.: Agricultural Research Service, U.S. Department of Agriculture, 1975)
and
Composition of Foods: Fruits and Fruit Juices, Agriculture Handbook No. 8-9, by Consumer Nutrition Center (Washington, D.C.: U.S. Department of Agriculture, 1982).

Page 65

"Vitamin C Gives Cancer Patients a Longer Life" adapted from "Supplemental Ascorbate in the Supportive Treatment of Cancer: Prolongation of Survival Times in Terminal Human Cancer," by Ewan Cameron and Linus

Pauling, *Proceedings of the National Academy of Sciences of the United States of America*, October, 1976.

Chapter 6

Page 77

"The Best Food Sources of Vitamin D" adapted from *Human Nutrition*, by Benjamin T. Burton (New York: McGraw-Hill, 1976).
and
McCance and Widdowson's The Composition of Foods, by A. A. Paul and D. A. T. Southgate (New York: Elsevier/North-Holland Biomedical Press, 1978).

Chapter 7

Page 83

"The Best Food Sources of Vitamin E" adapted from "Vitamin E Content of Foods," by P. J. McLaughlin and John L. Weihrauch, *Journal of the American Dietetic Association*, December, 1979
and
Nutritive Value of American Foods in Common Units, Agriculture Handbook No. 456, by Catherine F. Adams (Washington, D.C.: Agricultural Research Service, U.S. Department of Agriculture, 1975)
and
McCance and Widdowson's The Composition of Foods, by A. A. Paul and D. A. T. Southgate (New York: Elsevier/North-Holland Biomedical Press, 1978).

Page 84

"Vitamin E Boosts 'Good Guy' Cholesterol" adapted from "The Effect of Tocopherol on High-Density Lipoprotein Cholesterol," by William J. Hermann, Karen Ward and James Faucett, *American Journal of Clinical Pathology*, November, 1979.

Page 85

"Calf Cramps while Walking? Vitamin E Takes Them in Stride" reprinted by permission of the publisher from *Vitamin E: Biochemical, Hematological, and Clinical Aspects*, Bertram Lubin and Lawrence J. Machlin, eds. (New York: New York Academy of Sciences, 1982).

Chapter 8

Page 101

"The Best Food Sources of Calcium" adapted from *Nutritive Value of American Foods in Common Units*, Agriculture Handbook No. 456, by Catherine F. Adams (Washington, D.C.: Agricultural Research Service, U.S. Department of Agriculture, 1975).

Page 107

"The Best Food Sources of Potassium" adapted from *Nutritive Value of American Foods in Common Units*, Agriculture Handbook No. 456, by Catherine F. Adams (Washington, D.C.: Agricultural Research Service, U.S. Department of Agriculture, 1975)
and
Composition of Foods: Dairy and Egg Products, Agriculture Handbook No. 8-1, by Consumer and Food Economics Institute (Washington, D.C.: Agricultural Research Service, U.S. Department of Agriculture, 1976)
and
Composition of Foods: Poultry Products, Agriculture Handbook No. 8-5, by Consumer and Food Economics Institute (Washington, D.C.: Science and Education Administration, U.S. Department of Agriculture, 1979).

Page 110

"Noise Drowns Out Magnesium" adapted from "Interaction of Noise-Induced Stress and Mg Decrease," by Harmut Isling, *Artery*, volume 9, number 3, 1981.

Page 111

"The Best Food Sources of Magnesium" adapted from *Composition of Foods*, Agriculture Handbook No. 8, rev. ed., by Bernice K. Watt and Annabel L. Merrill (Washington, D.C.: Agricultural Research Service,

U.S. Department of Agriculture, 1975)
and
Composition of Foods: Dairy and Egg Products, Agriculture Handbook No. 8-1, by Consumer and Food Economics Institute (Washington, D.C.: Agricultural Research Service, U.S. Department of Agriculture, 1976).

Page 113

"A Natural Cure for Kidney Stones" adapted from "Four Years' Experience with Magnesium Hydroxide in Renal Stone Disease," by G. Johansson et al., *Magnesium Bulletin*, February, 1981.

Page 115

"The Best Food Sources of Iron" adapted from *Nutritive Value of American Foods in Common Units*, Agriculture Handbook No. 456, by Catherine F. Adams (Washington, D.C.: Agricultural Research Service, U.S. Department of Agriculture, 1975)
and
Composition of Foods: Poultry Products, Agriculture Handbook No. 8-5, by Consumer and Food Economics Institute (Washington, D.C.: Science and Education Administration, U.S. Department of Agriculture, 1979).

Page 119

"The Best Food Sources of Zinc" adapted from "Zinc Content of Selected Foods," by Jeanne H. Freeland and Robert Cousins, *Journal of the American Dietetic Association*, June, 1976
and
"Provisional Tables on the Zinc Content of Foods," by Elizabeth W. Murphy, Barbara Wells Willis and Bernice K. Watt, *Journal of the American Dietetic Association*, April, 1975
and
"Zinc and Copper Content of Seeds and Nuts," by Kenneth G. D. Allen, Leslie M. Klevay and Hugh L. Springer, *Nutrition Reports International*, September, 1977.

Page 123

"The Best Food Sources of Chromium" adapted from "Mineral Elements: New Perspectives," by Walter Mertz, *Journal of the American Dietetic Association*, September, 1980.

Page 125

"Selenium and Disease" map compiled from figures supplied by the U.S. Bureau of the Census and the American Cancer Society.

Chapter 10

Page 146

"Timed-Release: Its Timing Is Off" adapted from "Ascorbic Acid Absorption in Humans: A Comparison among Several Dosage Forms," by Susanna Yung, Michael Mayersohn and J. Barry Johnson, *Journal of Pharmaceutical Sciences*, March, 1982.

Page 149

"Synthetic and Natural Vitamin C" adapted from "Bioavailability of Synthetic and Natural Ascorbic Acid," by O. Pelletier and M. O. Keith, *Journal of the American Dietetic Association*, March, 1974.

Photography Credits

Cover—Margaret Skrovanek.
Staff Photographers—Christopher Barone: pp. 13; 15; 20; 22; 36; 47; 54; 70; 71; 73; 74; 108; 143; 148. Carl Doney: pp. 11; 26; 52; 76. T. L. Gettings: pp. 24; 150. John P. Hamel: pp. 31; 38; 61. Mark Lenny: p. 1. Mitchell T. Mandel: pp. 27; 51; 80; 82; 91; 100; 126; 130; 131; 133; 136; 144. Margaret Skrovanek: pp. 56; 79; 85; 90; 97; 112; 153. Christie C. Tito: pp. 63; 68; 103; 128. Sally Shenk Ullman: p. 58.

Other Photographers—Howard Hall: p. 141. Grant Heilman: pp. 3, 132. Maurice and Sally Landre: p. 102. Al Zalon: p. 33.

Additional Photographs Courtesy of—American Health Products Co., Inc., Orangeburg, N.Y.: p. 151. Coagulation Laboratory of Lehigh Valley Hospital Center, Allentown, Pa.: p. 86. John L. Gerin, Georgetown University: p. 28, center right. NASA Jet Propulsion Laboratory: p. 8. Freelance Photographers' Guild, New York: p. 121. Bruce Korant, DuPont Co., Wilmington, Del.: p. 28, top, center left and bottom. National Association for Sickle Cell, Los Angeles, Calif.: p. 95.

Illustration Credits

Bascove: pp. 2; 12; 23; 39; 41; 45; 48; 59; 77; 83; 92; 101; 105; 107; 111; 114; 115; 117; 119; 123; 137; 142. Susan Blubaugh: pp. 18; 29; 40; 50; 62; 64; 69; 89; 94; 122; 135; 140. Joe Lertola: pp. 5; 9; 14; 35; 42; 43; 44; 53; 55; 60; 65; 66; 78; 87; 99; 104; 110; 113; 118; 125; 129; 138-139; 155.

Index

A

Acidophilus, therapeutic value of, 128
Acne, effect of vitamins on, 24-25
Alcohol
    deficiencies due to, 27, 40-41, 51,
      59-60
    need for supplements with,
      11, 16-17
Alfalfa, therapeutic value of, 129
Allergies, need for vitamin C with, 59
Amino acids, therapeutic value of, 130-31
Anemia, 116. *See also* Iron deficiency
    in children, 119
    folate deficiency as cause of, 51, 52
    sickle-cell, vitamin E deficiency and, 95
Antihistamine, vitamin C as, 61
Antioxidants, 82-83
Arthritis
    effect of cod-liver oil on, 139
    relief of pain from, 92, 94, 107
    rheumatoid, 71, 121
    use of niacin for, 44
Atherosclerosis
    cause of, 84-85
    effect of insulin and chromium on, 122
    effect of lecithin on, 142
    effect of vitamin E on, 84-85

B

B complex vitamins, 37-55. *See also*
  specific vitamins
    how to buy, 149
Bee pollen, 132
Behavior
    effect of iron deficiency on, 117
    effect of vitamin B_6 on, 48-49
Beriberi, 2-5
Beta-carotene, 23, 148
    cancer and, 34
Bioflavonoids, 71-73
Biotin, 53, 55
Biotin deficiency, effects of, 55
Blindness, nutritional causes of, 26, 27
Blood pressure
    effect of magnesium on, 114
    effect of potassium on, 109-11
Bone
    calcium in, 98, 101
    health of, vitamin D and, 75, 77-78
Brewer's yeast, therapeutic value of, 133
"Buffered," definition of, 146
Burns, treatment for, 69-70, 135

C

Cadmium, 120
Cadmium toxicity, nutritional defense
  against, 19
Calcium, 101-4
    benefits of, 97, 103-6
    best levels of, 106-7
    effect of on bone, 98, 101-6, 151
    excess of, effects of, 161
    high blood pressure and, 98
    how to buy, 150-51
    importance of in colon, 79
    levels of, guidelines for, 161
    need for supplements of, 12
    RDA for, 108
    therapeutic dosages of, 161
    versus estrogen, 98
    vitamin D and, 75, 103

Calcium deficiency, effect of, 104-5
Cancer
    avoidance of, 34, 78-79
    beta-carotene and, 23, 34
    breast, 24, 124-25
    effect of selenium against, 9, 124-25
    endometrial, estrogen and, 102
    PCBs and, 31
    vitamin A and, 21, 23, 24, 34-35
    vitamin C and, 64-65, 67
    vitamin E and, 89, 94
Cataracts, 43, 82
Cell(s)
    effect of antioxidants on, 82-83
    importance of vitamin A to, 28-29, 34
    melanoma, effect of vitamin C on,
      67
    red blood. *See* Red blood cells
Charcoal, therapeutic value of, 134
Chelation, facts about, 147
Chlorophyll, therapeutic value of, 135
Cholesterol
    effect of brewer's yeast on, 133
    effect of calcium on, 105
    effect of chromium on, 123
    effect of lecithin on, 142-43
    effect of vitamin B_6 on, 46
    effect of vitamin C on, 67-69
    effect of vitamin E on, 84, 85-86, 150
    functions of, 67
Choline, 53, 54-55
Chromium, 121-23
    atherosclerosis and, 99, 122
    benefits of, 133
    blood sugar levels and, 122-23
Chromium deficiency, effect of, 123, 154
Circulation
    effect of bioflavonoids on, 72
    effect of calcium on, 106
    effect of vitamin B_6 on, 46
    effect of vitamin E on, 81
Cod-liver oil. *See* Fish-liver oil
Cold sores, relief of, 73, 128, 131
Colds, vitamin C and, 61-62
Contraceptives, oral, nutritional effect
  of, 11, 17, 47, 52
Cramps
    menstrual, effect of calcium on, 106
    muscle, calcium and, 104, 105, 106
      use of vitamin E for, 85, 94
Cysts, use of vitamin E for, 94

D

Demineralization of bones, vitamin D
  and, 75
Depression
    effect of phenylalanine on, 131
    folate deficiency as cause of, 52
    use of niacin for, 45
    vitamin B_6 deficiency and, 48
Desiccated liver, therapeutic value of, 136
Diabetes
    brewer's yeast and, 133
    effect of bioflavonoids on, 72-73
    effect of chromium on, 123, 154
    effect of vitamin E on, 87, 94
Dialysis, kidney, need for zinc with, 120-21
Diarrhea, relief of, 128, 134
Disease
    barriers against, vitamin A and, 28-29
    food as cure for, 1-9
Drugs
    effect of, on vitamin C, 57, 59, 63
      on vitamin B_{12}, 51
    need for supplements with, 17

E

"Emulsified," definition of, 146
Endometrial cancer, estrogen and, 102
Endurance, effect of vitamins and
  minerals on, 18-19
Energy
    effect of potassium on levels of, 111
    effect of vitamin B_6 on, 48
    importance of vitamin C to, 62
"Enzymes added," definition of, 146
Estrogen
    calcium versus, 98
    effect of, 17
    health problems linked to, 102
    use of for osteoporosis, 101-4
Evening primrose oil, therapeutic value
  of, 137
Exercise
    effect of, on cholesterol, 85
      on nutritional balance, 18
    need for riboflavin with, 18
    vitamin B_6 and, 48
Eyes
    riboflavin and, 43
    vitamin A and, 26-27
    vitamin B_6 and, 49
    vitamin E and, 83, 94

F

Fat(s)
    effect of on chromium levels, 99
    effect of alfalfa on, 129
    effect of lecithin on, 142
    effect of vitamins C and E on, 86
    role of in cancer, 124
Fatigue
    anemia and, folate deficiency as
      cause of, 52
    iron deficiency and, 116
    pantothenate and, 53
Fertility, effect of zinc on, 120-21
Fertilizers, synthetic, effect of on food,
  115
Fibrocystic breast disease, effect of
  vitamin E on, 94
Fish-liver oil, therapeutic value of, 7,
  138-39
Flatulence, effect of charcoal on, 134
Flu, vitamin C and, 62
Folate, 51-53
    effects of riboflavin on, 42
    excess of, effect of, 159
    levels of, guidelines for, 159
    therapeutic dosages of, 159
Folate deficiency, effect of, 51-52
Folic acid. *See* Folate
Food(s)
    absorption of iron from, 119
    disease and, 1-9
    effect of processing on, 15-16, 47,
      84, 109
    effect of synthetic fertilizers on,
      115
    junk, thiamine deficiency and, 40
Food supplements, need for, 11-19

G

Gallstones
    effect of lecithin on, 143
    effect of vitamin B_6 on, 46
Ginseng, 140
Glandulars, 140
Glaucoma, use of vitamin A to control, 27
Glucose tolerance, effect of chromium
  on, 122-23

Glycosides, 140
Gums, healthy, 70, 135, 136

H
Hay fever, pantothenate and, 53
Healing
    usefulness of minerals for, 98
    wound, 21, 89-90, 120, 123
Hearing, effect of vitamin A on, 25-26
Heart
    benefits of cod-liver oil for, 138-39
    brewer's yeast and, 133
    effect of thiamine on, 40-41
    effect of vitamin C on, 67-69
    effect of vitamin E on, 81, 84-87
    importance of minerals to, 98
    magnesium deficiency and, 111
Heat stress, effect of potassium on, 110-11
Herpes, relief of, 92, 128
High blood pressure, minerals and, 98
Hot flashes, use of vitamins for, 95
Hyperactivity, use of vitamin B$_6$ for, 49
Hypertension, effect of potassium and
    sodium on, 108

I
Immune system
    effect of diet on, 94
    effect of vitamin A on, 21, 27-29
    effect of vitamin E on, 81, 83-84, 94
    effect of zinc on, 119-20
    importance of vitamin C to, 60-61
Impotence, zinc and, 98
Infection
    effect of acidophilus on, 128
    effect of charcoal on, 134
    effect of vitamin C on, 60-61
    effect of vitamin E on, 95
    effect of zinc on, 119-20
    resistance to, 21, 116
Infertility, 21, 70-71, 98
Insomnia, 45, 106, 130
Insulin, effect of chromium on, 122, 123
Iodine, 25, 141
Iron, 115-19
    benefits of, 97, 117-18
    blockage of, 16
    excess of, effects of, 162
    levels of in average diet, 99, 115-16
        guidelines for, 118, 162
        riboflavin and, 42-43
    RDA for, 99
    therapeutic dosages of, 162
    vitamin C and, 59, 119
Iron deficiency, 116, 117-119

J
Junk foods, thiamine deficiency and, 40

K
Kelp, therapeutic value of, 141
Kidney stones, 49, 69, 113-14

L
Lead, nutritional defense against, 19,
    98, 114
Lecithin, therapeutic value of, 142-43
Leukemia, effect of vitamin C on, 61, 67
Leukoplakia, vitamin A and, 24
Lipoproteins, effect of vitamin E on,
    84, 85
Liver, 8, 23, 54
    effect of lecithin on, 142
    desiccated, therapeutic value of,
        136

M
Magnesium, 112-15
    effect of, 48-49, 112, 113-14
    excess of, effect of, 162
    high blood pressure and, 98
    levels of, 114, 115
        in average diet, 98-99
        factors affecting, 113, 114-15
        guidelines for, 114, 162
    noise stress and, 110, 113-14
    therapeutic dosages of, 162
Magnesium deficiency, effect of, 112-13
Mastitis, cystic, effect of vitamins on,
    24, 94
Melanoma cells, effect of vitamin C on, 67
Menstruation
    calcium and, 107
    vitamin A and, 21
    vitamin B$_6$ and, 47
Minerals. *See also specific minerals*
    absorption of, 98
    benefits of, 8-9, 18-19, 97-125
    chelated, 147
    deficiencies of. *See specific*
        minerals
    how to buy, 150-51
    importance of to health, 99
    levels of, 8, 14
    sources of, 8
    trace, 9
Mineral supplements
    how to take, 147
    need for, 15-19
Muscle cramps
    calcium and, 104-6
    vitamin E and, 94
Muscles
    effect of iron on, 116-17
    importance of potassium to, 110

N
Nerve(s)
    disorders of, use of choline with, 54
    effect of calcium on, 106
    effect of thiamine on, 38-40
    importance of vitamin B$_{12}$ to, 50
Neuralgia, relief of with vitamin E, 92
Niacin, 43-45
    benefits of, 44-45
    excess of, effects of, 157
    levels of, guidelines for, 157
    pellagra and, 2
    sources of, 2
    therapeutic dosages of, 157
Niacin deficiency, effect of, 44-45
Night blindness, vitamin A deficiency
    and, 26
Nitrates, levels of in body, 67
Nitrogen dioxide (NO$_2$), 31-32, 88
Noise, effect of on magnesium levels,
    110, 113-14
Nutrients
    body's need for, 11, 154
    factors that drain, 11-19

O
Oil, fish-liver, therapeutic value of, 7,
    138-39
Oral contraceptives, nutritional effect
    of, 11, 17, 47, 52
"Organic," definition of, 146-47
Osteoarthritis, vitamin E and, 92, 94
Osteoporosis, 75, 101-4, 151
Oxidation, effect of, 82, 86, 89
Ozone, 19, 63, 88-89

P
PABA. *See Para-aminobenzoic acid*
Pain
    arthritis, relief of, 92, 94, 106
    bone, effect of calcium on, 104-5, 106
    effect of niacin on, 44
    effect of tryptophan on, 130-31
    effect of vitamin E on, 92
Pantothenate
    benefits of, 53
    levels of, guidelines for, 159
    RDA for, 53
    stress and, 18, 53
    therapeutic dosages of, 159
Para-aminobenzoic acid (PABA), 53, 54
PCBs. *See Polychlorinated biphenyls*
Pellagra, 1-2, 43, 45
Pesticides, nutritional defense against,
    19, 63
Phenylalanine, 131
Phenylketonuria (PKU), 131
Phosphates, iron and, 16, 117
Phosphorus, importance of vitamin D
    to, 75
Platelet aggregation, effects of vitamins
    on, 46, 84, 87
PMS. *See Premenstrual syndrome*
Pollen, bee, 132
Pollutants, nutritional defense against,
    16, 19, 30-34
Pollution
    benefit of minerals against, 98
    effect of on nutritional balance, 11,
        19, 77
    effect of vitamin E against, 82, 88, 89
    effect of zinc against, 120
    need for vitamin C against, 63
Polychlorinated biphenyls (PCBs), 31, 63
Potassium, 107-8, 110
    effect of, 107-110
    heat stress and, 108, 110-11
    high blood pressure and, 98, 107-9
    levels of, 109-10
    loss of, 98, 107-8, 109
    sodium and, 107-8, 109
    sources of, 106, 111, 154
Pregnancy, nutritional needs during,
    43, 47, 52
Premenstrual syndrome (PMS), effect
    of vitamin B$_6$ on, 47
Pro-vitamin A. *See Beta-carotene*
Pyridoxine. *See Vitamin B$_6$*

R
Recommended Dietary Allowances
    (RDAs), 12, 14
Red blood cells
    effect of ozone on, 88-89
    riboflavin and, 42-43
    vitamin B$_{12}$ in production of, 50
Rheumatoid arthritis, relief of, 71, 121
Riboflavin (vitamin B$_2$), 41-43
    levels of, guidelines for, 157
    need for with exercise, 18
    red blood cells and, 42-43
    therapeutic dosages of, 157
Riboflavin deficiency, effect of, 41-42, 157
Rickets, 6-8, 75

S
Selenium, 99, 124-25
    benefits of, 9, 97, 98, 124-25
    harmful effects of, 9, 125
Selenium deficiency, effect of, 154
Serotonin, 39, 130
Shingles, use of vitamin E for, 92

Sickle-cell anemia, vitamin E deficiency and, 95
Skin
    effect of riboflavin deficiency on, 42
    effect of vitamin A on, 21, 24-25, 91
    effect of vitamin C on, 70
    effect of vitamin D on, 91
    effect of vitamin E on, 83, 90-92, 93
Skin infection, use of charcoal for, 134
Smog, vitamin E and, 87-89
Smoking, effect of on nutritional balance, 18, 59, 63
Sodium
    effect of on hypertension, 108
    potassium and, 107-8, 109
Sore throat, effect of chlorophyll on, 135
Sores, cold, relief of, 73, 128, 131
Spasms, effect of calcium on, 105-6
Sperm
    effect of vitamin C on, 70
    effect of zinc on, 120
Stamina
    effect of iron deficiency on, 116
    effect of vitamin B$_6$ on, 48
Steroids, effect of vitamin C on, 63
Stress
    benefit of minerals during, 98
    effect of, 11, 18, 30
    effect of desiccated liver on, 136
    effect of magnesium on, 113-14
    effect of pantothenate on, 53
    effect of vitamin A on, 21, 30
    effect of vitamin C on, 59, 63-64
    effect of vitamin E on, 87-89
    heat, effect of potassium on, 110-11
Strontium, 99, 141
Sugar
    blood, effect of vitamin E on, 87
    effect of on chromium levels, 99, 123
    milk, intolerance to, 128
Sunlight
    effect of on bone growth, 7, 75
    importance of to vitamin D levels, 8, 78-79
Supplements
    individual program for, 145, 153-63
    mineral, how to take, 147
    need for, 11-19
    shopper's guide to, 145-51
    special, evaluation of, 127-43
Surgery
    vitamin A and, 29
    vitamin B$_{12}$ and, 51
    vitamin C and, 71
    vitamin E and, 87
    zinc and, 98, 120

T
Taste
    effect of zinc on, 121
    need for vitamin A for, 26
Temper, effect of calcium on, 105
Tension
    menstrual, effect of vitamin B$_6$ on, 47
    neurotic, effect of thiamine on, 40
Thiamine (vitamin B$_1$), 38-41
    beriberi and, 5
    levels of, guidelines for, 156

loss of, 3-4, 14, 41
    therapeutic dosages of, 156
Thiamine deficiency, effect of, 39, 40-41, 156
"Timed-release," definition of, 147
Trace amines, 131
Trace minerals, 9
Tranquilizer
    niacin as, 45
    tyrosine as, 131
Tryptophan
    effect of, 130-31
    niacin and, 45
Tumors
    breast, effect of vitamin A on, 24
    effect of arginine on, 131
    formation of, effect of antioxidants on, 83
    levels of vitamin E with, 83
Tyrosine, tranquilizing effect of, 131

U
Ulcers
    effect of chlorophyll on, 135
    effect of vitamin E on, 90
    effect of zinc on, 120

V
Vision
    night, 27, 121
    sharp, importance of vitamin A to, 21
Vitamins. *See also specific vitamins*
    B complex. *See* B complex vitamins
    benefits of, 13, 18-19, 53
    deficiencies of. *See specific vitamins*
    levels of, in average diet, 14
    loss of, 15-19
    natural versus synthetic, 147-48
    timed-release, effectiveness of, 147
Vitamin A, 21-35
    as defense against toxic chemicals, 19, 21
    benefits of, for eyes, 21, 26-27, 83
      for skin, 21, 24-25, 91
    effect of lecithin on, 142
    effect of zinc on, 121
    emulsified, 146
    excess of, 22, 156
    how to buy, 148-49
    levels of, in average diet, 22-24
      guidelines for, 22, 23, 156
Vitamin A deficiency, 23
    causes of, 28
    effect of, 26, 27, 29, 156
Vitamin B$_1$. *See* Thiamine
Vitamin B$_2$. *See* Riboflavin
Vitamin B$_6$ (pyridoxine), 45-49
    benefits of, 46-49
    effect of on energy, 19, 48
    excess of, effects of, 158
    levels of, guidelines for, 158
    therapeutic dosages of, 158
Vitamin B$_6$ deficiency, effect of, 11, 46-47
Vitamin B$_{12}$, 49-51
    levels of, guidelines for, 50-51, 158
    therapeutic dosages of, 158
Vitamin B$_{12}$ deficiency, 50-51
Vitamin B$_{15}$, 55

Vitamin C, 57-73
    as defense against chemicals, 16, 19, 63
    benefits of, 24, 60-62, 64-65, 67-71, 86
    buffered, definition of, 146
    effect of drugs on, 59-60, 63
    excess of, effects of, 160
    how to buy, 149-50
    iron and, 59, 119
    levels of, guidelines for, 59, 160
      RDA and, 58-60, 69
    loss of, 15-16, 18
    therapeutic dosages of, 160
    timed-release, effectiveness of, 146
Vitamin C deficiency, effect of, 57, 69
Vitamin D, 75-79
    bone health and, 75, 77-78, 103
    effect of lecithin on, 142
    effect of, 78-79, 91, 138
    emulsified, 146
    excess of, effect of, 77, 160
    levels of, guidelines for, 77, 160
    RDA for, 76
    sources of, 77, 138
    synthesis of, 8, 76-77
    therapeutic dosages of, 160
Vitamin D deficiency, effect of, 7, 75-76
Vitamin E, 81-95
    benefits of for skin, 25, 83, 90-92, 93
    blockage of lead absorption by, 19
    cancer and, 83, 89, 94
    effect of, on cholesterol, 85-86, 150
      on circulatory system, 81, 84-87
      on immune system, 81, 83-84, 94, 95
    emulsified, 146
    how to buy, 150
    levels of, guidelines for, 84, 88, 161
    pollution and, 82, 88, 89
    RDA for, 83
    therapeutic dosages of, 161
Vitamin E deficiency, effect of, 86, 87, 95
Vitamin K deficiency, effect of vitamin E on, 161
Vitamin supplements, need for, 15-19

W
Wounds
    healing of, chromium and, 123
      vitamin A and, 21
      vitamin E and, 89-90
      zinc and, 120

X
Xerophthalmia, 27

Y
Yeast, brewer's, therapeutic value of, 133

Z
Zinc, 119-21
    benefits of, 9, 98, 119-21
    effect of, 8, 121
    excess of, effect of, 163
    how to buy, 151
    levels of, in average diet, 99
      guidelines for, 163
    RDA for, 99
    therapeutic dosages of, 163
Zinc deficiency, surgery and, 120

Rodale Press, Inc., publishes PREVENTION®, the better health magazine.
For information on how to order your subscription,
write to PREVENTION®, Emmaus, PA 18049.